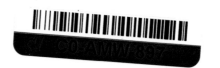

RELIGION THAT HEALS, RELIGION THAT HARMS

To Dusty,

With warm regards,

[signature]

8-22-10

RELIGION THAT HEALS, RELIGION THAT HARMS

A Guide for Clinical Practice

James L. Griffith

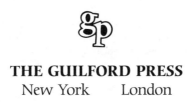

THE GUILFORD PRESS
New York   London

To Lynne, whose fierce love keeps me forever in the field of play

*To my late father, Lamont Griffith, who showed me
that person-to-person relatedness is neither preceded by a "why?"
nor followed by an "in order to"*

*In memory of Tom Andersen, Michael White, and Harry Goolishian,
whose lives and work created a radical humanism
in which everything about a person in psychotherapy would be pushed back,
so the person could be fully brought forward*

© 2010 The Guilford Press
A Division of Guilford Publications, Inc.
72 Spring Street, New York, NY 10012
www.guilford.com

Printed in the United States of America

This book is printed on acid-free paper.

Last digit is print number: 9 8 7 6 5 4 3 2 1

Library of Congress Cataloging-in-Publication Data

Griffith, James L., 1950–
    Religion that heals, religion that harms : a guide for clinical practice /
James L. Griffith.
        p. ;   cm.
    Includes bibliographical references and index.
    ISBN 978-1-60623-889-9 (hardcover : alk. paper)
    1. Mental illness—Religious aspects.   2. Mentally ill—Religious life.
3. Psychology, Religious.   I. Title.
    [DNLM: 1. Psychotherapy—methods.   2. Religion and Psychology.
3. Mental Disorders—psychology.   4. Mental Disorders—therapy.
5. Professional-Patient Relations.   6. Sociobiology.   WM 420 G853r 2010]
    RC455.4.R4G76 2010
    616.89—dc22
                                                        2010019292

About the Author

James L. Griffith, MD, is Professor of Psychiatry and Neurology and Associate Chair of the Department of Psychiatry and Behavioral Sciences at the George Washington University Medical Center in Washington, DC. He also is Director of the Psychiatry Residency Program and Director of the Psychiatric Consultation–Liaison Service in George Washington University Hospital. As an educator, Dr. Griffith has developed a program of psychiatric residency training that balances biological and psychosocial therapies in the treatment of patients within their family, community, and cultural contexts. His first book, *The Body Speaks: Therapeutic Dialogues for Mind–Body Problems* (1994), introduced family-centered approaches for treating psychosomatic disorders and psychosocial sequelae of chronic medical illnesses. A second book, *Encountering the Sacred in Psychotherapy: How to Talk to People about Their Spiritual Lives* (2002), presented a clinical approach for incorporating the spiritual and religious resources that patients bring to clinical settings. Currently, Dr. Griffith provides psychiatric treatment for immigrants, refugees, and survivors of political torture at Northern Virginia Family Services in Falls Church, Virginia. From 2000 to 2004, he served as Director of Training for the Kosovar Family Professional Educational Collaborative, a project to develop a family-centered mental health system in Kosovo. Dr. Griffith has received the Human Rights Community Award from the United Nations Association of the National Capital Area and the Margaret B. and Cyril A. Schulman Distinguished Service Award from the George Washington University Medical Center, for both the training of mental health professionals and the development of mental health services in the Washington metropolitan area for survivors of political torture; Psychiatrist of the Year from the Washington Psychiatric Society; and the Distinguished Teacher Award from the George Washington University School of Medicine.

Preface

I EMBARKED ON WRITING THIS BOOK 5 YEARS AGO. I SENSED the need for a fresh clinical approach to addressing religious and spiritual issues in health care, one that could more even-handedly promote salutary effects of religious life while countering adverse ones. This need was pressing at a distinct juncture in the history of the relationship between religion and medicine. The last decades of the 20th century witnessed a resurgence of interest by clinicians in the role of religion and spirituality in health. As the century closed, regular workshops on spirituality in health care were offered in many clinical disciplines; curricula on spirituality were incorporated into the educational programs of medical schools and postgraduate residencies; and, for mental health clinicians, a plethora of textbooks and clinical trainings on spirituality were available. In 2002 Melissa Elliott and I authored *Encountering the Sacred in Psychotherapy* as a textbook for psychotherapists seeking to incorporate patients' spiritual resources in their psychotherapies. Most of these efforts, as did our text, shared common aims of respecting patients' religious identities and utilizing their spiritual lives as resources for healing and resilience. Done less well, however, was assessment and intervention for problems that have long been common knowledge but seldom discussed: how religion can harm as well as heal, and damage as well as protect.

My awareness of destructive uses of religion drew from both personal and professional recollections. Over the 38 years of my medical career, I remember the cases where no one seemed able to help because a patient had become so sequestered by religious beliefs that he or she could not trust clinicians or accept needed treatments. My psychiatric work with medically ill patients brought me into regular contact with those whose religiousness motivated suicide, violence, or neglect of health needs, or led to unnecessary exacerbations of suffering. In my personal life, I knew both acquaintances and kin who abandoned relationships or hurt others needlessly out of some dispute over religious beliefs. Like many, I have been repeatedly puzzled by the strange disconnect between some persons' religious beliefs that saluted love and compassion while their actions fueled hatred and violence, all the while feeling no conflict between the two. For clinicians, there was little specific guidance other than to take charge forcibly when someone appeared at risk for serious harm, turning a doctor–patient relationship into a police action.

To some extent, advocacy for religion and spirituality has stood in the way of serious efforts to address their dark sides. Religion has long carried the stigma of being antiscience within modern medicine, and antagonism toward religion within psychiatry and psychology has been at times vitriolic. Clinicians seeking a broader incorporation of patients' religious lives in coping with illnesses have been hesitant to join criticisms of religion's harmful potential for fear that their words might be twisted by religion's enemies. This, however, is only a partial explanation. Melissa Elliott and I in fact devoted our longest chapter in *Encountering the Sacred in Psychotherapy* to "When Spirituality Turns Destructive." I nevertheless realized at the time of its publication and in a subsequent journal article (Griffith & Griffith, 2002, *Journal of Family Psychotherapy*, 13[167–194]) that our efforts had fallen short of what clinicians needed. In retrospect, this was the only possible outcome. We were utilizing narrative theory and cultural symbology for our theoretical underpinnings: how one can use idioms, metaphors, stories, beliefs, dialogues, and other symbolic forms when conducting psychotherapy with a religious person. Such an approach can be richly generative when utilizing spirituality within a context of dialogue to promote healing and resilience. It offers little, though, for addressing destructive uses of religion, most of which operate outside contexts of dialogue. Destructive uses of religion in fact originate largely outside language in behavioral systems shared with other mammals. People using religion destructively rarely sit down with a psychotherapist to examine and reflect upon their actions.

This book turns to two different scientific domains—neurobiology and sociobiology—for a conceptual framework and clinical methods that can address what goes terribly wrong when religious life produces suffering rather than relieves it. Further into the text, this social neuroscience is joined with observations from existential philosophers whose phenomenological methods arrived at similar destinations from different starting points. Above all, this is a clinical textbook that seeks to provide a reader with a clinical map and accompanying methods for assessing and intervening effectively when religious life threatens to harm a patient or others within the patient's life space. Its aim is to distinguish that which is healing and protective in religious life, while countering that which can be damaging. Although this volume focuses on religion's destructiveness, it should be read as a complement to *Encountering the Sacred in Psychotherapy*, a textbook that illustrates manifold ways for psychotherapies to draw from a person's religious life to support solace, healing, and resilience.

It is fair to ask an author to disclose his or her personal beliefs and religious point of view so they can be taken into account in the reading. Passions stirred by religion easily infiltrate a scientist's reasoning or a writer's text. Too much on religion and health has been published as "science" that, absent rigorous methodology, simply validated an investigator's prior religious, or antireligious, sentiments. Too much has been written by clinical teachers too uncritical of the extent to which their observations were shaped by their starting religious, or antireligious, assumptions. In *Encountering the Sacred in Psychotherapy*, I told in some detail my personal story and the development of my religious life (Griffith & Griffith, 2002, pp. 7–10). That account, however, said little about my history of affiliations with different organized religious groups or religious traditions. This text focuses upon actions that are influenced by beliefs and practices of religious groups. I should then disclose more about my history of allegiances to different religious groups.

Beginning with Southern Baptist churches in Mississippi, my religious journey has included membership and active participation in United Methodist, United Church of Christ, and Lutheran churches, as well as a Catholic lay fellowship, over the span of my adult life. At times I have served leadership roles, such as church elder. At present, I am a member of the Episcopal Church, an affiliation with which I am comfortable due both to the Episcopal Church's advocacy of progressive social causes and to the little harm it has done in the world, at least since the dissolution of British imperialism. Such a listing of churches, however, provides only markers, not a story. My journey through different spiritual traditions was not conducted randomly.

A growing commitment to action, rather than commitments to specific doctrinal beliefs, has guided my spiritual development since early adolescence. This included a changing attitude about religious beliefs and how obligatory their importance is in religious life. In contrast to the fundamentalist religious faiths of my youth, the quality of one's relatedness to other people—listening, acknowledgment, empathy, compassion, acts of mercy or protection—seemed so much more important than any particular propositional truths about God or Ultimate Reality. Systematic theology seemed a distraction from living. During medical school, for example, my participation in Wells Methodist Church in Jackson, Mississippi, was largely due to its location in an economically depressed and racially mixed neighborhood. Under the leadership of Reverend Keith Tonkel, Wells Church was providing city leadership toward racial reconciliation during the tense years of desegregation in the South. It conducted a free health clinic in its basement that provided health care for uninsured people, where I was in fact robbed at gunpoint one evening by consumers who wanted goods other than health care. Later, contact with Trappist monks whom I met during the Vietnam antiwar movement led to a year of weekly instruction in Catholicism and a near-decision to join the Catholic Church. My decisions to join one church or another increasingly reflected my appraisal of how much difference they were making in their neighborhoods and society. Otherwise, my formal religious participation in adulthood has drifted steadily toward the liturgical. I suppose it is the physical, nonverbal aspects of the Catholic and Episcopal masses—the kneeling, the ritual of the Eucharist, the space for silence—that have innately drawn me to them.

I recently reread Thomas Merton's *Contemplative Prayer* and recognized a strong kinship with Merton's experience of religious faith. Whether or not I would have shared his theology, it seems I have traversed territory of like kind in my own life, making similar observations and bearing similar thoughts, although in secular arenas far from Gethsemane Monastery. In *Contemplative Prayer*, written shortly before his death, Merton speaks about "wordless contemplative prayer in purity of heart, without images or words, even beyond thoughts" (1969, p. 56), and contrasts this with discursive prayers spoken in full sentences or communal prayers of a body of worshippers. Such impulses of the heart and wordless prayer, mostly points of awareness of intimate contact with self, God, and others, now make up most of my religious life. Speaking in such terms possibly would merit classification as "mystic" in Karen Armstrong's (1993, pp. 395–397) schema of religious life. Suffice it to say that I have never encountered a theology or religious system that did not put distance between me and that which I encounter as the Divine. Since I don't expect my experience of living necessarily to extend to others, I try as best I can to acknowledge the different experiences of others and their validity. I strive to stay curious and interested in how others experience religious life differently. This is the personal vantage point from which I write and conduct my clinical work. While these sentences may not answer all questions a reader might pose about my religious experience and perspective, I hope they will indicate that I come with no ideology to proclaim and seek no followers to lead. My work should speak for itself.

A second concern for a reader might be the range of an author's exposure to the world's religious faiths other than the Christian culture of North America. Here the answer is more complex. My personal religious history of course has been solidly within the American Protestant and Catholic Christian religious traditions, with degrees of exposure to Judaism. However, I have studied Islam, Buddhism, Hinduism, and some other religious traditions. I have taught professionally through lectures, workshops, and seminars in 20 countries, many of which have been Muslim cultures of the Balkans, Persian Gulf, and Africa. Last year I spent the final 2 weeks of Ramadan with a dozen Saudi physicians in North Africa, joining them as they broke fast in the evenings, watching with them the televised ritual readings of the Qurán in Mecca and Medina, celebrating Eid, engaging in endless discussions of Islam, Judaism, and Christianity. More important, my psychiatric practice has been focused on immigrants, refugees, and political torture survivors in the Washington metropolitan area, for whom their spiritualities often have been critical in recovering lives from trauma, loss, and violence. My patients and their Buddhist, Sikh, Hindu, and Muslim psychotherapists, counselors, and case managers have taught me about illness and health in the contexts of their religious faiths. My expertise and exposure to the world's faiths has been uneven, but it has been broad.

This leads to an obvious question: Why are there so many Christian patients in the vignettes of this book? Many vignettes, in disguised form, are drawn from the medical, surgical, and psychiatric services of George Washington University Hospital in Washington, DC, one of our nation's most culturally and ethnically diverse cities with a large representation of many of the world's religions. Internists and surgeons requesting psychiatric consultation are usually preoccupied with the clinical problem—a patient refusing treatment or threatening suicide—without prior awareness of the patient's religious identity. I am skeptical that a religious mix of patient populations, case selection, or clinician bias taken together can adequately explain why there is a preponderance of Christian cases in the vignettes of this book. These observations lead to questions that this book can raise but cannot answer: Are some religious traditions more at risk than others for harm? Or, put more specifically, does the personalization and anthropomorphizing of a Deity that characterizes the Christian faith also open specific risks for harm to self or others? These are potentially answerable questions for empirical researchers from the psychology of religion, but beyond the scope of this text to settle.

This book is dedicated to Lynne Gaby, my colleague and wife. Lynne stayed steadfast in her conviction that I should write, turned our best bedroom into my study, and slept alone in the midnight to 3:00 A.M. hours when I found the stillness that the work required.

It is also dedicated to my late father, Lamont Griffith, at whose bedside the last words of this text were written shortly before his death. My father refused to be subdued by the physical disabilities from his World War II head injury and neck fracture. He showed how to play the hand that life deals without bitterness or resentment, to face what comes, to press forward relentlessly. Above all, he showed how to draw energy from person-to-person relationships, unsullied by rank or class.

This book is dedicated as well in memory of three family therapy clinicians whose innovations made possible my work. Were they now living, Michael White, Tom Andersen, and Harry Goolishian each might be baffled to find this dedication in a textbook about religious patients. Yet each helped create a radical humanism that is a bedrock therapeutic stance from which to conduct psychotherapy. Their ideas and values created a culture out of which the pages of this book were written. They each would embrace a person embracing a religiously determined life, however alien that life might have been for them personally.

Other people also made essential contributions to the writing. Jim Nageotte, my editor at The Guilford Press, has been constant in speaking to my strengths, helping me see the vision of my work, and extending however much time it needed beyond our starting projections. Conversations with Jim always pushed the ideas down good paths that I would not have found on my own. Jeff Akman, my departmental chair at George Washington University, has been masterful in building a psychiatry department that is financially sound, hence relevant within our institution, while also sustaining an academic culture whose humanist commitments value such clinical work as that articulated in this text. Such departments can be rare in American psychiatry of our era. Finally, John Gualtieri, psychologist and psychotherapist, helped me channel my deep passions into creating and writing. The back story to this book is that I was awakening in the middle of the night during the 2004 presidential campaign too enraged to sleep. Christians were beating their plowshares into swords. Religious beliefs and biblical scriptures that in my youth were simply tools for compassion were being turned into political knives of hatred against gays and lesbians and anyone else deemed outside the fold of Christianity-as-ideology. This disruption took me back to psychotherapy, which in turn led to a decision to write this book. It would be a professional book with little chance to undo corruption of religion in broader society, yet would tackle the problem within a sector where I had expertise: the worlds of medicine and psychiatry.

The clinical concerns of this text bridge multiple professional communities. Where possible, "clinician" is used as an inclusive and generic term for professional consultants that include psychiatrists, psychologists, social workers, nurses, family therapists, and licensed professional counselors, while acknowledging its inadequacy as a descriptor for chaplains and clergy. More problematic has been finding an inclusive term for persons at the center of clinical problems, where "patient," "client," "parishioner," and "consumer" are identity flags for different professional communities that also speak to different therapeutic traditions and practices. Lacking a more universal term, I have used "patient" as describing best not only the language but the character of professional relationship in the clinical vignettes. The Greek etymology of "patient" as "to suffer" is at the heart of identity in these stories. I was a doctor treating patients, from my perspective and theirs, in my clinical encounters.

Protection of personal identity is a challenge when writing about patients' lives. In order to instruct with validity, clinical vignettes must closely follow the contours of real-life interactions with real people. Placing clinical fiction in a professional book that guides actions of clinicians toward real patients is dangerous. Yet too close a description violates a commitment to confidentiality implicit in all therapeutic relationships. To avoid these pitfalls, I have followed common practices of clinical authors by altering identifying information—gender, ethnicity, age, profession, and other markers—in order to disguise personal identities. Sometimes I have blended factual descriptions drawn from different clinical encounters of similar kinds across my years of practice as a physician and medical school professor.

Contents

When Religion Goes Bad
A Mental Health Problem?

MS. JOHNSON HAD GONE THROUGH HER FOURTH SURGERY IN
5 months after cancer was diagnosed. Concerned about her depressed mood,
her surgeon asked me for a psychiatric consultation. My evaluation, however,
found few hallmark signs of depression. Rather, the patient was demoralized
and lonely, as anyone might be, as a result of the physical debilitation of her
illness, her concerns about her children at home, and the unreliability of her
husband's emotional support. When I entered her room, I had noticed an
open Bible at the head of Ms. Johnson's bed. I listened to her description
of the past 5 months of struggle and then asked, "From where do you draw
strength to get through a time like this?"

"God and my friends," she responded. She told how she read the passages from the Bible repeatedly. She also prayed and attended a neighborhood
church.

I asked what was her favorite verse of scripture. She paused and then
answered, "By his stripes I am healed."

"When I hear you mention that verse," I commented, "it makes me think
that you must know that God feels your pain."

Ms. Johnson then began weeping and told how dwelling upon God's caring had, in fact, lessened her pain. She did not think she would have been able
to endure the stress of her illness without God to rely upon.

Ms. Johnson's story is a common one. Many people who live with illnesses—physical or mental—do so by resting upon a faith in and a relationship with a personal God. However, not every story of God and illness is as edifying.

Mr. Lankton, an elderly 62-year-old man, was on renal dialysis following complications from cancer treatment. Psychiatric consultation was requested after he had been found bleeding profusely with his dialysis access catheter pulled loose. The nurses were unsure whether this was an accident or intentional. For some time Mr. Lankton denied any awareness of what had happened. Well into the interview, he made an odd comment regarding worries he had about the nurses outside in the hall. As I pressed for details, he finally said, "I'm afraid they will bleed to death." I realized then that he was psychotic, unable to distinguish his internal world from the external one around him, and projecting his fears onto the nurses. When I asked whether he ever worried that something like that could happen to him, he abruptly asked if we could pray together. I agreed, provided that he lead the prayer. He began by praising God and thanking God for all the blessings of his life. Then he said, "Dear God, please help the doctors to understand that when you call someone to be with you in heaven, they need to stand aside." Like Ms. Johnson, Mr. Lankton also relied upon his faith in and his relationship with his God. However, this faith, influenced by psychotic thinking, was now driving him to suicide.

Religion Presents Moral Dilemmas

The sway that religion holds over human life can be enormous. Unfortunately, religion has just as much power to impose suffering on human life as it does to alleviate suffering. Much like atomic energy, which can make either bombs or electricity, religion is not good or evil but simply powerful. People who mobilize humanitarian responses to war or famine often do so as an expression of their religious faiths. Yet religious conflict often helped cause the war or famine in the first place. Religious faith can move a person to risk his or her life to protect an unknown stranger. Yet religion can serve as justification for killing one's neighbors when they do not share one's religious identity. As psychology of religion researcher Lee Kirkpatrick has commented (2005, p. 5):

> The idea that religion is broadly "good" or "bad" is absurd on its face: Like
> virtually any aspect of human experience and behavior, it no doubt is both
> in myriad ways (and neither in other respects). It seems patently obvious

from thousands of years of human history that religion can be a powerful force in promoting either peace or war, mental health or mental illness, prosocial or antisocial behavior, racism or universalism, happiness or misery.

Among those who bear debilitating illnesses, some attribute their survival primarily to their religious lives. For others, however, religious life has deepened despair, obstructed access to needed treatment, or justified a life-threatening neglect of one's health. Examples are easy to find to argue that religion is either humankind's greatest gift or its greatest curse.

Exacerbating Illness and Suffering: Religion's Dark Side

This moral duality of religion is a practical concern for clinicians who witness the influences of religion in their patients' lives. Religious beliefs and practices powerfully impact how people perceive, think about, and respond to the problems for which they seek clinical treatment. For many, these religious influences are health promoting, but for some they are not. A few examples—and these do not exhaust the list—underscore this point.

Ms. Ames, a 56-year-old African American woman, was admired by her colleagues for her professional accomplishments despite the racial discrimination and poverty of her childhood in the Old South. Now, however, she had fallen inexplicably ill. Suddenly and without warning, she would lose awareness of her surroundings, fall to the ground, and begin jerking her arms and legs uncontrollably. She could not safely drive her car and was beginning to question whether she should leave her job because of medical disability. Standard regimens of anticonvulsant medications were of no help in stopping the seizures. Eventually, Ms. Ames was hospitalized in a sophisticated epilepsy diagnostic center where her seizures could be videotaped while her brain electrical activity was continuously monitored. This evaluation produced a surprising finding: Her seizures did not come from epilepsy at all. Rather, they were entirely a stress-induced behavioral disorder. A psychiatric consultation then disclosed a different story of her illness. As a child, Ms. Ames had been physically abused by her alcoholic father and had regularly watched her mother being beaten as well. Like many survivors of childhood abuse, she carried a long-term vulnerability into her adult life with a body perpetually poised for alarm whenever there was even a trace of conflict. Angry voices or arguing would trigger this alarm. When severe, exposure to conflict led to a dazed state and seizure-like jerking of her arms and legs.

The current precipitant of Ms. Ames's symptoms was her marriage. Her husband, who had progressed little in his career, felt belittled when his work life was compared with his wife's public recognition as an attorney. With a low threshold for frustration, he would berate her relentlessly. The tirades sometimes went on for hours, while she tried to placate him. Ms. Ames believed the marriage had been a mistake. Her friends advised her to divorce. However, she also believed an earthly marriage was eternal. As a Christian, she believed divorce could not be considered an option. She tried to persevere, keeping the verbal abuse hidden, even as her seizures had worsened. The steadfastness of her religious faith became an active agent in producing her illness.

Ms. Ames's story eventually ended well. She accepted her neurologist's and psychiatrist's findings about the nonepileptic origins of her symptoms. She began noting and reflecting upon the connections between her seizures and the emotional agitation she felt when her husband vented his anger. She prayed about her dilemma. Her spiritual focus gradually shifted from a fear of sinning against her church's teachings to viewing her seizures as "a wake-up call from God," meaning she needed to make her health a top priority or else it would be taken from her. She utilized her psychotherapy to navigate separation and divorce from her husband. With an ending of her marriage, her seizures stopped entirely. She began a new life with renewed zest, feeling supported both by her religious faith and by her family, friends, and clinicians.

By contrast, the story of Mr. Chin had a more troubling ending. Mr. Chin, an elderly, warm-faced Chinese man, had fractured his femur in a fall and now was refusing surgery. Although he would likely survive without surgery, he would have to live with a shortened leg, chronic pain, and walking only with an assistive device. A psychiatric consultation was requested to determine whether Mr. Chin had the capacity to refuse the surgery. In discussing with Mr. Chin the surgeon's recommendations, it was quickly evident that he understood the medical facts of his injury, why surgery was recommended, and the risks if he refused it. It was also clear that he had no psychiatric disorder affecting his thinking. Rather, he reasoned thoughtfully within his belief system. Mr. Chin was a member of the Fulan Gong religious faith. He wanted to rely upon his meditative spiritual practices, his religious faith, and the support of his Fulan Gong community to bring about his physical healing. He showed me some of the Fulan Gong religious literature, which was replete with dramatic first-person testimonies of people who had recovered from dreaded and hopeless medical diseases through faithful adherence to the Fulan Gong way. Mr. Chin had clung tenaciously to his faith during years of persecution by the Chinese government before emigrating to the United States. In his elder years, he did not wish to depart from the beliefs and practices of the Fulan

Gong that had long defined his identity. After a lengthy interview aided by a Mandarin-speaking translator, I concurred that Mr. Chin had the capacity to make his medical decisions, including a refusal of surgery. His request to be discharged to the care of his Fulan Gong community was granted.

Sometimes religious issues do not directly speed the progression of disease, yet do add unnecessarily to its misery. Ms. Dylan was a young woman with multiple sclerosis. Psychiatric consultation had been requested for treating her depressed mood. As we spoke, her level of distress was immediately evident. Yet she did not have symptoms of a pervasive mood disorder, as do many multiple sclerosis patients. Her mood, in fact, was scored in the normal range on a quantified scale for assessing depression. Noting the guilty tone in which she spoke about her illness, I asked Ms. Dylan whether she ever felt it was a punishment. She nodded and revealed that she had been promiscuous as a teenager. She believed all things that happened in her life occurred under God's dominion: "If you do something wrong, you are punished," she was taught as a little girl. Now she believed that she had been afflicted with multiple sclerosis as God's punishment for her behavior. I told her I viewed this differently but understood how this could be her belief. If she did believe it though, did she also believe there was a way the punishment could be lifted? "By prayer and asking forgiveness," she responded. I asked whether she had prayed. "I haven't prayed in a long time, because I feel God is angry with me." "Are you afraid to pray?" I asked. "Yes, with everything I've done, I don't have the right to pray."

I met jointly with Ms. Dylan and her psychotherapist to explain why I felt an antidepressant would not be helpful. I recommended that they make the breakdown of relationship between Ms. Dylan and her God a focus of their work, hoping that this could open a different resolution to her making sense of her illness.

The stories of Mr. Lankton, Ms. Ames, Mr. Chin, and Ms. Dylan are revisited later in this text. For now, I simply note that each of their religious faiths, which one might hope would help them traverse life's struggles, instead was exacerbating illness and suffering. Helping them with their clinical problems meant responding to these adverse impacts of their religions.

Listening for the Unannounced Influences of Religion

The influences of religion in health care are often ignored. They commonly lie offstage, in the background of a clinical encounter, omitted from the stories that clinicians recount about their patients. The significance of religious faith was paramount in each of these vignettes, yet evident only after a specific inquiry sought its significance.

Seldom does a person present a religious problem as a clinical concern, even when a religious issue is at the center of a treatment failure. Of the prior four cases, only Mr. Chin's situation was cast from the start as involving a religious issue. However, religious commitments often contribute to impasses in medical or psychiatric treatment.

Clinical problems in which religious issues are often embedded include refusal of needed medical or psychiatric treatments, physical or emotional abuse, coercion or violence, impulses to suicide, neglect of physical hygiene or health needs, and social isolation. These are often clinical emergencies because someone's safety—often the patient but sometimes another person— is at risk. There is every reason to believe that Mr. Lankton would have ended his life had he been given the opportunity. More often, the issue is not one of safety but an unnecessary exacerbation of personal suffering, sometimes tragically so.

More mundanely, religion can motivate attitudes and habits that affect health. Religious beliefs and practices often affect the timing for when someone seeks treatment, whether there is trust and openness with clinicians, and whether clinicians' directives are followed. Ms. Johnson's religious faith sustained her confidence in her surgeons and their treatment protocols past the point where repeated disappointments might have led her to give up. However, Mr. Chin's religious faith led him to refuse treatment by his orthopedic surgeons, who possessed the medical expertise to repair his broken hip.

Religion also affects health by shaping a person's social space. This often bolsters health. Research studies, for example, have shown a correlation between church attendance and good health (Koenig et al., 1997). Church attendance itself may or may not have direct effects on good health. However, those who attend church have less exposure to people who smoke cigarettes, abuse drugs, drive recklessly, or get into bar fights. Omission of these behaviors from one's social space can be a potent contributor to good health. On the other hand, a strong religious identity can render a person uniquely vulnerable to social predators who select religious groups within which to operate. As has been repeatedly witnessed in religious cults, fundamentalist faiths, and other tightly knit groups, religious leaders can use the language and garb of faith to manipulate, exploit, and abuse those who trust them.

Less certain, but plausible, is the role of religious experience in altering the body's physiological processes. Research in psychosomatic medicine has documented how negative emotions—despair, loneliness, resentment, helplessness, shame, guilt—can activate processes of disease as a result of deleterious effects upon the body's endocrine, immune, and autonomic nervous systems (Harris & DeAngelis, 2008; Mookadam & Arthur, 2004; Koenig, 1998). Certain medical diseases are particularly sensitive to exacerbation by physiological changes associated with negative emotions. Moreover, nearly any psychiatric disorder can be activated by negative emotions sustained too intensely for too long. Although one would hope that religious faith would attenuate such negative emotions (Koenig et al., 1997), it sometimes is the case that religious faith amplifies them. Although there has been little formal research on adverse physiological effects from specifically religious factors, there are reasons for concern when religion becomes a chronic generator of negative emotions in the life of a medically ill or mentally ill person, as when a person experiences exaggerated guilt for personal sins, believes illness to be a punishment from God, or feels abandoned by God in a crisis. (Pargament, Koenig, & Tarakeshwar, 2001, 2004).

Most Destructive Consequences of Religion Are Not Due to Mental Illnesses

Physical and emotional abuse, coercion, violence, risky health behaviors, neglect of self, social isolation, exaggerated despair, physiological stress symptoms—on the face of it, all these might seem to be markers for psychiatric illnesses. However, this is usually not the case, as discussions in Chapters 5, 6, 7, and 8 detail. Religious behaviors that harm people most often express complex sociobiological behaviors that in many contexts might be protective or simply have no bearing on health. Sociobiological systems for attachment, peer affiliation, kin recognition, social hierarchy, and social exchange are discussed as some examples of these. When religion turns destructive, usually one or more of these sociobiological systems has come to overshadow a person's capacity to respond as a whole human being to the needs of self or others. For example, religious behaviors that facilitate identification with one's religious group can also extinguish a sense of accountability to those outside the group. Religious beliefs can create such a totalizing, all-encompassing picture of "what is real" that everything within its purview is defined, ordered, and assigned meaning, to the exclusion of any alternatives. Religious practices that make one's life feel coherent and purposeful can violate a felt sense of connectedness to those who do not adhere to the same beliefs and practices. Sociobiological processes that enable a religious group to feel cohesive and its members to feel competent can also propel violence toward others, particularly when

personal empathy is weak across the group boundary. Clinically, it is important to understand sociobiological patterns through which harm can occur
without overmedicalizing them as mental illnesses. These patterns point to
clinical interventions that can overlap with, but are often distinguished from,
those used to treat mental illnesses.

Some Destructive Consequences of Religion Are Due to Mental Illnesses

Religion sometimes is little more than a voice for psychiatric symptoms. Psychiatric symptoms can be as easily conveyed by religious discourse as by music,
art, writing, or other modes of human expression. Moreover, strong emotions
stirred by religion, particularly those of vulnerability, uncertainty, and threat,
can be potent activators of mood, anxiety, and psychotic symptoms. Religious
zeal can sometimes trigger the onset or exacerbate the intensity of psychiatric
illnesses.

When religion interacts with psychiatric illness, the levels of complexity
multiply. Religious beliefs color a person's thoughts, feelings, and behaviors
with an added hue of meaning. When a person already is depressed, religious
beliefs can irrationally amplify guilt, apathy, or self-hatred. Religious beliefs
can escalate the intensity of intrusive thoughts in obsessive–compulsive disorder. Religion that activates a sense of uncertainty or dread can intensify any
anxiety disorder. As with Ms. Ames, religious beliefs that silence expression
of felt distress can set the stage for somatization and medically unexplained
physical symptoms. Religion can transform delusions and hallucinations in
dramatic and destructive ways among patients with schizophrenia or other
psychoses. Religious beliefs have lethal consequences when used to justify
suicidal or homicidal impulses. Those with psychiatric disorders suffer daily,
often in ways hidden to others around them, and religious faith sometimes
exacerbates this suffering instead of lessening it. Chapters 9, 10, 11, and 12
examine how a patient's religious life can interact with mood, anxiety, and
psychotic disorders.

Should Health Professionals Address Destructive Consequences of Religion?

There has been long-standing controversy over the role of clinicians in the
religious lives of their patients. One can build a multilayered argument that
a person's religious life bears strongly upon physical and mental health, often

for good but sometimes for ill. However, does that mean it is the business of a health care professional to intervene in religious life?

Cogent arguments have been posed for keeping a strict boundary between a patient's religious life and the professional competencies of clinicians. Most of these have been put forward as ethical concerns on behalf of the patient's autonomy. Respect for autonomy means treating a patient as someone who can deliberate about personal goals and be guided by those deliberations. This means giving priority to a patient's opinions, values, and choices, stepping back from imposing the clinician's values upon the patient (Beauchamp & Childress, 2001).

Richard Sloan, a professor of behavioral medicine at Columbia University (Sloan, Bagiella, VandeCreek, & Poulos, et al., 2000; Sloan, 2006, 2007), has been a leading critic of efforts to integrate the healing methods of spirituality and religion into health care (Koenig, 1998; Miller, 1999; Puchalski, Larson, & Lu, 2001; Sperry & Shafranske, 2005). He has emphasized three ethical concerns about clinicians who encourage their patients to engage in religious practices. First, the clinician–patient relationship is an unequal one in regard to its distribution of power. There is an implicit expectation that clinicians prescribe and patients comply with treatment. It is thus difficult for a clinician to "suggest" religious activity, such as praying for a healing recovery, without this becoming coercive. Second, there are many other factors that unequivocally have an impact on health (e.g., cultural, political, economic) and yet are considered to lie outside the province of a clinician's expertise. Marriage, for example, might be protective for the health of an elderly man who lives alone with multiple chronic medical illnesses. However, most would deem it inappropriate for his physician to prescribe marriage. Third, there is the possibility of doing harm. Interventions into the moral lives of people are not neutral. Encouraging a patient to focus on his or her religious life plausibly could strengthen coping, but it also could do harm if the patient were to conclude in despair that the medical illness had been inflicted by God as a punishment.

These critiques are all valid concerns. Too often physicians and other healers have failed to monitor either personal hubris or ideological zeal in making recommendations that ended with harmful consequences for patients. However, reasonable responses can be made to each of these concerns short of a call for clinicians to exit the religious lives of their patients. First, it is true that there is a paucity of scientific evidence for the usefulness of any particular religious belief or practice when prescribed as treatment, be it prayer, attending church, or studying sacred scriptures. However, an enormous body of research points to harmful health effects from such emotional states as confusion, despair, helplessness, and loneliness. Less robust but still substantial is research pointing to protective effects from such positive states as hope, optimism, and a sense of connection and emotional support from others (Harris & DeAngelis, 2008; Taylor & Gonzaga, 2007; Uchino, Holt-Lunstad, Uno, Campo, & Reblin, 2007). At the least, the research of psychosomatic medicine supports a clinical role for helping patients find effective ways to utilize their spiritual resources—their own, not the clinician's—toward sustaining states of positive emotions.

Sloan's comparison of religion to marriage, in fact, points to an appropriate role for a clinician. There is little evidence that marriage engenders health when society as a whole is considered. In fact, two early research studies found marriage to predict an earlier death among breast cancer patients (Waxler-Morrison, Hislop, Mears, & Kan, 1991; Ell, Nishinoto, Medianslay, Montell, & Hamovitdh, 1992). However, subsequent research studies have shown that it is the quality of the marital relationship that is the "active ingredient" with effects on health, for good or bad (Hibbard & Pope, 1993, Weihs, Enright, & Simmens, 2008). Competent clinicians can appropriately and favorably influence the quality of either marriage or religion in patients' lives. This role is an easy fit for mental health professionals whose professional practices already are spent traversing the landscapes of their patients' emotional and relational worlds.

Second, mental health clinicians are not experts on religion, yet they do have professional skills for addressing problems involving communications, relationships, and the roles of values and beliefs in a person's life. Competent mental health clinicians have training that can address these aspects of religious life while still respecting a patient's autonomy.

Third, there are indeed risks of harm when interventions involve a patient's religious life, but this is also true of every medical treatment. What matters more is the attention given to the underlying ethical principles of patient autonomy and clinician beneficence: benefits for the patient must be maximized and risks minimized, with the patient given informed consent about choices (Beauchamp & Childress, 2001). An increasingly large clinical literature argues that trained mental health professionals can work collaboratively with a patient to address *how* religious experiences affect health and well-being, without specifying *what* beliefs and practices are valid (Blass, 2007; Galanter, 2005; Griffith & Griffith, 2002; Josephson & Peteet, 2004; Pargament, 2007; Puchalski et al., 2001).

Some critics have argued that clinicians are too ill equipped to address religious issues competently or too unable to avoid intrusions of their personal religious ideologies into professional duties. Their solution has been to erect a wall that keeps clinicians' hands off the religious lives of their patients.

This book supports these ethical concerns but takes a different tack: to try to understand mechanisms through which religion's underside can do harm, to distinguish these from mechanisms that can be healing, and to devise clinical strategies through which clinicians can address patients' religious lives in both their healing and harmful aspects.

The approach proposed in these pages utilizes sociobiology and neurobiology to make harmful uses of religion intelligible. These perspectives can strengthen a practitioner's hand in devising contexts for dialogue with religious patients who might otherwise eschew contact with a mental health clinician. The aim is conversation within which both clinician and patient find voice, seeking solutions free of coercion but responsive to both the clinician's concerns and the patient's religious commitments. This strategy establishes a committed posture toward dialogue despite power asymmetries in the clinician–patient relationship.

Clinicians Challenged
by Religiously Determined Patients

Religiously determined patients can alarm their clinicians with their actions toward selves or others. Often the double meaning of "determined" is fitting, in that religion determines the patient's identity and the patient determines to impose a religious stamp upon the clinical encounter. Broadly, mental health professionals are responsible for learning how spirituality and religion impact the health of those whom they treat. Specifically, they should command the skills needed to interact with religiously determined patients in a manner that is respectful, compassionate, and clinically responsible.

Assessment of probable health effects of a person's religious beliefs and practices can be incorporated into the usual diagnostic evaluations that clinicians conduct. Such an assessment can guide interventions that maximize salutary effects and minimize harmful ones, while respecting the person's religious identity and cultural traditions. This clinical role differs from the faith-based roles of clergy and chaplains by its primary reliance on the human sciences in understanding how religion and health interact. It makes best use of a clinician's "outsider" role as one who does not have a faith-based stake in how a patient conducts religious life but does wish to reduce suffering and promote health. From this outsider position, a clinician can ask questions with concern, respect, and authenticity. A clinician, without dictating or prescribing how to be religious, nevertheless can help a patient to become a more capable moral agent in his or her religious life.

Moving Beyond Conflicts over Behaviors: Rehumanizing Relationships with Religiously Determined Patients

Disputes over overt health behaviors can drive conflicts between clinicians and religiously determined patients. At odds, clinicians and patients may know each other only in hostile terms of refusals and defiance. Personal warmth and mutuality characterizing therapeutic relationships at their best are often casualties. Clinicians and patients are reduced as persons to positions in an argument.

When debate turns to dialogue, clinicians and patients conversely find that they can preserve vital identities and commitments while listening attentively to the other's reality. In dialogue the other is touched at a distance. There is more to aim for than simply brokering agreements about which behaviors will hold sway. What might a religiously determined patient need to heed in what a scientifically based clinician has to say? Do religiously determined patients bear messages to which clinicians need to attend? Where common ground in beliefs and behaviors cannot be found, can concern, compassion, and respect nevertheless find expression?

Beyond resolution of conflicts over religious behaviors, finding person-to-person relatedness in encounters between clinicians and religiously determined patients is a final aim of this book. The task is to expand the domain of dialogue when totalizing perspectives of clinicians and their religiously determined patients interlock. Sociobiology and neurobiology can help this expansion of dialogue through the fresh perspectives they offer. When dialogue is unachievable, sociobiological and neurobiological perspectives still can sharpen empathy, support compassion, and facilitate expressions of respect.

I

A Map for Navigating the Terrain of Religion

THE DUAL FACE OF RELIGION—RELIGION THAT HEALS, religion that harms—reveals itself not only in abstract theological debates, but also in intimate human encounters within hospitals, clinics, and psychotherapists' offices where patients and their families struggle with the adversities of illness. Nonobligatory suffering, self-neglect, treatment refusal, suicide, and violence each can be driven forward by a dark energy from religion. How to respond to these quandaries has been a longstanding challenge for secular clinicians. Religion defined by its themes of personal spirituality often becomes a bulwark, protecting emotional and physical survival for those who suffer. When religion takes a destructive turn, however, it usually has become coopted by one or more of the sociobiological systems that organize social life, or it is simply a megaphone for psychiatric illness. The first challenge for a secular clinician is how to open a conversation successfully about the role of religious life in coping. When this has been accomplished, neurobiological and sociobiological perspectives on religious life can further guide the clinical encounter to good ends by asserting the centrality of personal spirituality, while curtailing influences of sociobiology or mental illness, so that a patient can tap the benefits but avoid the pitfalls of religious coping.

1

✦

What Sociobiology Explains
about Destructive Uses of Religion

RELIGION AS BOTH BLESSING AND CURSE—HOW DOES ONE
respond to both faces of religion as a mental health professional? How should
one regard a patient's religious life when its clinical effects might be good,
bad, or irrelevant? A clinician, in fact, can help a patient to become more
competent and effective in making moral decisions within religious life, with
the patient rather than the clinician taking the guiding role. Helping patients
reach good decisions about "right" and "wrong" is not a role that mental health
professionals have historically relished, however. Psychiatry and psychology
originated in part through clinicians' efforts to distance themselves from the
moral discourse of religion. From a zone of moral neutrality, psychotherapists
from Sigmund Freud to B. F. Skinner have sought to bring science to bear
upon problems of humanity.

Nevertheless, a clinician can learn how to enter a patient's world in which
actions are about good and evil, right and wrong, guilt and atonement, sin and
forgiveness, in addition to the more familiar constructs of perceptions, cognitions, feelings, behaviors, and roles. Experiences of moral obligation, ethical
responsibility, and sense of justice can become part of clinical conversations.
A clinician can address this moral discourse within an intimate inquiry that
is enabled by skilled listening, well-crafted questions, and a therapeutic presence that stops short of taking over a patient's decision making. A clinical
map is needed to navigate this territory successfully.

Three Missions of Religion Exist in Uneasy Union

Risks of harm in religious life are to a great extent embedded in core roles that people most want religion to serve for their lives. Three of these roles are particularly salient in understanding how religion leads to healing effects in some instances and yet to harm in others. These three roles are interconnected but also distinct and separable. First, religion can help ensure group security, whether the group is a religious one or a neighborhood, ethnic group, or nation. Second, religion can strengthen the morale of individuals, supporting a sense of self as worthy and competent. Third, religion can attenuate personal suffering, for self or others. On the surface, these three missions may seem closely related. They do often coexist in harmony. However, they rely on fundamentally different processes, which creates fault lines across which they sometimes pull in opposite directions. Like the states comprised by old Yugoslavia, their surface tranquility disappears when too stressed, and they can tear apart at the seams.

These three missions of religion have different origins. Ensuring group security and building morale of individuals serve to mobilize sociobiological behavioral systems that originated through processes of biological evolution. The ascendancy of *Homo sapiens* over other early hominids depended upon cohesive social groups enabled by these behavioral systems. The role of religion in relieving personal suffering appears to have originated differently as a creative product of self-reflection and ethical decision making by intuitive and visionary religious leaders, a process shaped by dialogue, rhetoric, and other processes of cultural change, not biological evolution. To keep this distinction clear, the roles of religion in providing group security and morale of individuals are discussed as "sociobiological religion," while the role of religion in alleviating personal suffering is discussed as "personal spirituality."

Religion as a Quest for Group Security

Seeking safety within a strong group accounts for one of the initial thrusts of religion in human life (Barnes, 2003). If *Homo sapiens* held one decisive advantage over other early hominids, it was our species' capabilities for banding together in intelligently organized social groups for the common good (Mithen, 1996). Throughout history, religion has provided strong glue for the roles and responsibilities that make groups cohesive.

The readiness with which people sacrifice their individual lives out of loyalty to religious groups stands as one line of evidence for its importance.

Sixteenth-century Huguenots in France endured torture rather than betray their Protestant faith, while Catholics across the English Channel were suffering similar fates at the hand of their Protestant rulers. Death was considered to be a worthy price to pay for loyalty to one's particular brand of Christianity. Similar commitments have been regularly witnessed throughout history, from Jews dying in Russian pogroms and German concentration camps, to Muslims persecuted in Christian societies, to Tibetan Buddhists tortured by Chinese Communists, to American Mormons killed by American Protestants. Today many still place their lives at risk by putting forward their religious identities in settings of political conflict.

Religious group loyalty also can turn internally perverse. Too often, loyalty to one's religious group has led individuals to violate the most basic principles of morality. Religiously devout southern Christians from my Mississippi youth were silent for generations about racism and racial hate crimes that occurred regularly in their midst. Similarly, the religious today within Islam, an inclusive and tolerant religious faith, struggle to voice challenges against those who use the Qur'an and the Hadith to justify indiscriminate violence. Closer to home, confusion and anguish have run deep in the Catholic Church over revelations about pedophile priests who were protected for decades by their church leaders, who were aware of ongoing abuses of children. Examples of moral blindness of religious persons arising out of protective loyalty toward one's religious group occur so commonly as to seem mundane were it not for their awful consequences.

Religion as a Quest for Morale

Morale refers to one's sense of competence as a person. Possessing good morale means that a person feels capable of meeting one's own and others' expectations (de Figueiredo, 1993; Frank, 1961). Although morale is felt as an individual, it often is more a reflection of the status of one's group in society and one's status within that group (Tajfel, 1981; Pratto, Sidanius, Stallworth, & Malle, 1994). Personally, morale reflects confidence in oneself as an independent, autonomous person. Morale can be impacted at either level, externally by one's standing as a group or team member or internally via personal competencies supporting a sense of self.

Frank and Frank (1991) have reviewed evidence from a broad range of sources that an episode of demoralization is the usual antecedent for religious conversion or initiation into a religious cult. For example, Kildahl (1972) found more than 85% of tongue speakers to have experienced a personal cri-

sis preceding their speaking in tongues. This crisis typically involved feelings of worthlessness and powerlessness. The glossolalic experience invariably
resulted in a heightened sense of confidence and security.

Evangelical religious leaders and groups typically proselytize by deliberately exacerbating a targeted person's demoralization and then offering religious conversion as its solution. Sermons on guilt and damnation of the soul
are followed by an offer of grace and salvation. In daily life, religion is more
likely to be invoked in unusually stressful times than in response to more
mundane stressors. For example, Pargament (1997) has reviewed evidence
that people are more likely to pray over catastrophes and health crises than
such minor stressors as problems in the workplace. There is thus substantial
evidence that religion, like psychotherapy, can serve a major role in supporting personal morale (Griffith & Dsouza, in press).

The quest for morale can have its dark side. Religious practices that generate hatred toward those outside one's own group seem to bolster morale as
efficiently as, and perhaps more so, than religious practices that generate compassion. Sense of purpose, power, and ingroup camaraderie flow from moral
contempt expressed toward nonbelieving outsiders. These processes can contribute to what Marc Galanter (1999) has termed the "relief effect," an upward
surge in morale that new recruits often experience after joining a cohesive
religious group.

Religion as a Quest for Cessation of Suffering

According to the legend of the four passing sights, the father of Siddhartha
Gautama sought to protect him from the world's suffering by providing an
idyllic childhood where he would not witness human suffering. On a road,
however, Siddhartha encountered an old man, a diseased man, and a corpse
on a bier (Noss, 1963). After reflecting on this suffering, he devoted his life to
discovery of a path that could relieve other people of such an obligation. After
years of searching, he concluded that all life is suffering, we suffer because we
desire, and salvation resides in renouncing all desires, cares, or attachments.
Buddhism thus emerged as perhaps the purist of the world's great religions in
its single-minded focus on management of personal suffering.

Most other religions have not embraced so fully the path of renunciation
of desire in order to escape suffering. However, each has provided methods,
roles, and ideologies designed to build resilience against life's inevitable sorrows. A Muslim may thus experience suffering as God's test of one's character and faith, which then mobilizes the effort and energy needed to prevail
against the suffering. Christians' beliefs have ranged from viewing suffering as

God's just punishment, to believing that suffering contains God's hidden purposes, to feeling an assurance that God will provide sufficient strength to bear whatever suffering that life brings, to identification with Christ as a suffering servant. Each religion provides maps for navigating life's suffering, buffering its intensity, and mounting a coping response.

Unfortunately, there are myriad ways through which striving for deliverance from suffering propels religious behaviors that have untoward consequences. To the extent that one withdraws from the material world in order to reduce suffering, efforts to solve practical problems within one's society can cease, thereby augmenting suffering for others over the long term. Violence toward self by ascetics, or toward others by zealots, too often is committed in an expectation of gaining God's favor through obedience and sacrifice.

Religion Unequally Yoked in Its Missions

Religion can bring harm to peoples' lives when one or more of these three missions for group security, individual morale, and relief from suffering is prioritized selectively to the others' neglect. Usually such a split occurs when group security and morale building are each prioritized, but by straying from a mission to relieve suffering. The converse also seems to hold. Personal spiritualities with a singular focus upon alleviation of suffering usually pose few risks for harming individuals but may be ineffective in strengthening, and can even undermine, security of the group.

A clinician's professional mandate is sometimes to cure disease but always to relieve suffering. A clinical strategy for countering destructive uses of religion can support all three roles of religion in the good they can do. However, it must attend to their relative influences on patients' moral decision making and how those decisions play out in their real-life impacts on health or illness, comfort or suffering. An ethical clinician generally should not support or oppose any particular religious beliefs or practices. However, a clinician can help a patient to become a competent, effective moral agent in the decision making of his or her religious life, electing choices that best support health and most alleviate suffering, for self and for others.

What Do the Words "Religion" and "Spirituality" Mean?

"Religion" and "spirituality," unfortunately, are words that have become time worn, overburdened by layers of definitions and redefinitions by theologians and scholars, yet their use seems unavoidable because there are no good alternatives. Within the psychology of religion, empirical research has begun examining differences between spirituality and religion in how people use them in their lives. Hood, Hill, and Spilka (2009, p. 9) have summarized for the psychology of religion a current perspective:

> A traditional distinction exists between being "spiritual" and being "religious" that can be used to enhance our use of both terms. The connotations of "spirituality" are more personal and psychological than institutional, whereas the connotations of "religion" are more institutional and sociological. In this usage, the two terms are not synonymous, but distinct: Spirituality is about a person's beliefs, values, and behavior, while religiousness is about the person's involvement with a religious tradition and institution.

Hood and his colleagues emphasize that spirituality has more to do with the interior psychological lives of individuals, while religion is more manifest in group life and society as a whole. The discussion in this book incorporates similar horizons of meaning, while focusing on pragmatic and clinical effects of religion and spirituality as both are enacted in people's lives.

But Does "Spirituality" Pass the Nazi Test?

An additional criterion needs inclusion in definitions of spirituality: Can one's description of spirituality pass the "Nazi Test"? In an October 4, 1943, speech to SS Group Leaders in Poznan, Heinrich Himmler summarized Nazi morality in the Third Reich:

> One principle must be absolute for the SS man: we must be honest, decent, loyal, and comradely to members of our own blood and to no one else. What happens to the Russians, what happens to the Czechs, is a matter of utter indifference to me. Jewish Virtual Library (n.d.)

Can a particular definition of spirituality distinguish between Mother Theresa and Heinrich Himmler? That is, does it help distinguish between someone whose purpose and commitment are anchored in compassion for society's excluded and exploited and someone whose meaning and commitment are anchored in exclusion and exploitation of those outside one's group of identity? If the difference appears obvious, it often isn't.

Generally, definitions that primarily characterize spirituality as a source of ultimate meaning or connection have trouble passing the Nazi Test. In recent years, many have sought to separate spirituality from formal religion by regarding spirituality in more personal terms as one's source of meaning and purpose in living or one's sense of connectedness with others, so much so that nearly anything providing meaning and connection can count as "my spirituality." In educating physicians, the Association of American Medical Colleges recently announced its support of medical school curricula about spirituality and health, considering spirituality to be "an individual's search for ultimate meaning through participation in religion and/or belief in God, family, naturalism, rationalism, humanism, and the arts" (Association of American Medical Colleges, 1999, pp. 25–26). Putting spirituality in such terms of ultimate concerns, deep sources of meaning, or positive emotions is certainly inclusive of most spiritual traditions. However, such definitions have difficulty distinguishing between saints and demons when both are drawing energy from sources greater than themselves.

Two themes of personal spirituality best discriminate it from ideological "isms": a commitment to person-to-person relatedness independent of any social categorization and an ethic of compassion that extends to all persons, even those outside one's own religious or social group. Other prominent themes of spiritualities discriminate less well. It is possible to live a life of devotion to God, derive purpose from sacred teachings, find fellowship with other believers, and devote oneself selflessly to religious group missions, all the while showing indifference, or even hatred, toward those who not belong to one's religious group or share in a common religious identity. Awareness of and responsibility for the well-being of those on the outside best discriminates personal spirituality from other powerful social processes, religious and nonreligious, that also provide existential meaning and sense of connectedness with others. The Nazi Test focuses attention upon the quality of relatedness with those who live outside one's group. Spirituality embraces persons, not categories. Spirituality extends human relatedness to those not observant of one's own beliefs and practices or who do not belong to one's spiritual community. Religiousness is not spirituality when it sets relationships by first distinguishing whether a person is "one of our own."

Separating personal spirituality from religious or ideological zeal is critical. My personal recollections of these differences often have been poignant. As a concrete example, a classmate in high school was a member of the Ku Klux Klan. His conversations were an even blend of Biblical scriptures and White supremacy, all worked out in a logically tight ideology. He, in fact, put me to shame with his religious devotion. His dreaminess, conviction, and joy in talking about a society that would protect our racial purity made it obvious that he would fight, perhaps even die, for his beliefs. How would this be different from any of Jesus's disciples who died martyrs' deaths?

Over the years I have met other dreamy ideologues who were Jewish, Muslim, or Hindu, as well as from a variety of Christian sects, each restricting empathy and compassion to their own religious group. Making the distinction between personal spirituality and religious zeal became a pragmatic concern as I began working professionally in multicultural settings that juxtaposed many different ethnic and religious groups. The problem, it seemed, was that religion could uplift, energize, and fortify individuals for life's struggles through multiple pathways whose superficial similarities belied deep differences. One pathway, sociobiological religion, was made available through the ideology, roles, responsibilities, and hierarchy of one's religious group. A different pathway, personal spirituality, became available instead through emotional relatedness between individuals who, person to person, touched each others' lives in the uniqueness of their beings.

Using a Sociobiological Lens to Untangle the Confusion of Religious Life

Religion describes a wide and messy swath of human life instead of a cohesive and singular factor that bears consistent effects upon people. Sociobiology and evolutionary psychology provide tools that can render religion more comprehensible by unraveling some of its complex psychological and social effects.

Sociobiology consists of the interdisciplinary efforts by biologists, sociologists, ethologists, anthropologists, and archaeologists to explain complex social behaviors in terms of evolutionary advantages that particular behaviors may have held for early human species (Wilson, 1978). Evolutionary psychology, an offshoot of sociobiology, has studied the origins of human intelligence, including such social capacities as the ability to make psychological sense of another person's thoughts, feelings, or intentions (Mithen, 1996). Evolutionary psychologists have demonstrated how religion is expressed via multiple sociobiological behavioral systems (Kirkpatrick, 2005).

Sociobiological systems are compartmentalized behavioral systems that evolved according to the principle of inclusive fitness in order to solve specific survival problems faced by early hominids from 200,000 to 2 million years ago (Mithen, 1996). These sociobiological systems are fully operative today and organize how humans structure their groups and interpersonal relationships. As such, they both express and shape religious life. Sociobiological systems that are particularly salient in religious life include those for attachment, peer affiliation, kin recognition, social hierarchy, and social exchange.

Attachment: "God Is My Good Parent."

The attachment system evolved to ensure that mothers and their offspring would bond securely and protectively. Within the brains of mammals, the attachment system is organized to guide motivational, emotional, and memory processes with respect to significant caregiving figures. Children and parents are each driven to seek closeness with each other when alarmed or insecure (Siegel, 1999). The attachment system governs person–God relationships as well.

At the end of World War II, John Bowlby (1973) originally conceptualized attachment theory to explain the different patterns of distress shown by children who had been separated from their parents during the London blitz. Bowlby identified as key elements of the attachment system: (1) "proximity," as a child seeking nearness to a primary attachment figure; (2) "secure base," as a child's playing and exploring with ease only when a primary attachment figure is close at hand; and (3) "safe haven," as a child seeking out a primary attachment figure when feeling threatened or insecure. When God is an important attachment figure, these themes of proximity, secure base, and safe haven are lived out in relationship with one's personal God.

Whereas the attachment system among other mammals is based only upon physical proximity to a parent, human attachments are organized around the felt presence and emotional responsivity of a caregiver (Bowlby, 1973). In an attachment relationship, one's thoughts, feelings, and behaviors are largely oriented toward that relationship. Early attachment to parents or other primary caregivers becomes internalized into an enduring attachment style that reflects attitudes about relationships, their importance, and how they ought to be managed. If early life attachments are problematic, absence of a sense of secure base can produce an attachment style organized by insecurity, with impaired play, exploration, and social interactions (Siegel, 1999).

For many religious people, God is one of their most important attachments. Kirkpatrick (2005, p. 52) has noted that "the perceived availability and responsiveness of a supernatural attachment figure is a fundamental dynamic underlying Christianity and many other theistic religions. Whether that attachment figure is God, Jesus Christ, the Virgin Mary, or one of various saints, guardian angels, or other supernatural beings, the analogy is striking." In his studies of different kinds of prayer, Hood, Spilka, Hunsberger, and Gorsuch (1996, p. 394) have noted how some types of prayer seem preoccupied mainly with the responsivity of God rather than petitioning God to intervene on one's behalf through actions. For example, contemplative prayer is an attempt to approach and to relate deeply to one's God, and meditative prayer mainly reflects concerns about the quality of one's relationship with God.

People with insecure attachments to their Gods can be more vulnerable to demoralization when adversity strikes. A secure attachment to a personal God can act as a potent buffer against demoralization, even substituting for failures in human relationships where attachments may be insecure (Griffith & Dsouza, in press; Rizzuto, 1979).

Peer Affiliation: "I Feel Secure as a Member of My Religious Group."

Like wolves and dogs, human beings appear hardwired to seek security as a member of a pack. Unlike other mammals who are limited to gestures and displays, humans can use language to signal desire for togetherness. Religious beliefs, rituals, ceremonies, and other practices commonly enable a sense of belonging to a group.

Peer affiliation refers to the bonds of brotherhood and sisterhood that usually do not carry the intensity or constancy of maternal attachment, but are more flexible, transient, and exchangeable. Peer affiliation is about relatedness by social category, roles, responsibilities, and loyalty to one's group. Religious identification often serves as a medium that facilitates cooperation, encouraging alliances and coalitions among those who share a common identity.

Drawing from his research on cult membership, Marc Galanter (1999) has articulated a theory of religion based on human needs for group affiliation. Religious groups are typically characterized by social cohesion so that personal circumstances of individuals are interlinked closely with other group members. There are shared concerns throughout the group. In cults, this social cohesion is intense, extending to uniform manners of dress, idiosyncratic language, and joint ownership of material possessions. Such mutuality fosters reciprocal altruism through which group members give freely to each other, assured that the same generosity will be given in return. For many, a church, synagogue, temple, or mosque is their key social network. Ken Pargament (1997) has detailed the many different ways in which people provide mutual social support within their religious groups.

A person who joins a cult often has felt debilitating loneliness and demoralization prior to joining. As mentioned earlier, Galanter's (1999) clinical research found in members of religious cults a reciprocal relationship between the lowering of precult anxiety and depression symptoms and the rise of social cohesion within the group, the "relief effect." This finding is further supported by social identity theorists who have documented the importance of memberships in national and ethnic groups for individuals' self-regard (Kirkpatrick, 2005).

Peer affiliation thus appears able to protect morale in the face of adversity. However, the strength of peer affiliation can depend on management of a firm boundary between those in the religious group and others outside it. This has unfortunate consequences when this boundary becomes a barrier to empathy toward those outside, justifying stigma, or in worse cases, coercion, exploitation, or violence.

Kin Recognition: "My Religious Group Is a Family That Looks Out for Its Own."

A social group must manage its boundaries with the outside world in order to survive. If there is no way to recognize who is or is not a group member, then the group ceases to exist. Religious groups appear to rely on kin recognition mechanisms that became components of human sociobiology eons ago. Neural circuits that underpin kin recognition operate at fundamental levels to discern biological features among family members, such as facial contours or smells (Daly & Wilson, 2005). The social processes of religious groups seem able to recruit these neural systems by evoking the experience of "family" through family metaphors and such descriptive language as "brother," "sister," and "father" applied to group members. Crippen and Machalek (1989, p. 74) described religion as a "hypertrophied kin recognition process" in which "kin recognition mechanisms are 'usurped' to form communities of fictive kin" (p. 68), which, in turn, encourages "individuals to subordinate their apparent self-interest to the collectively-expressed interest of sovereign agencies" (p. 70). Kirkpatrick (2005, p. 249) has noted that religious beliefs represent "a kind of cognitive error in which psychological mechanisms misidentify unrelated in-group members as kin, in much the same way that our taste-preference mechanisms can be fooled into enjoying soft drinks or potato chips flavored with artificial sweeteners and fat substitutes."

Shared religious language and practices can thus define an ingroup, with ingroup members receiving privileges and respect not afforded to those in outgroups. Fundamentalist religions are largely about establishing and defending an ingroup that is defined by specific beliefs and practices, relegating those who do not observe them to outgroup status. Fundamentalism is thus a form of religion in which coalitional psychology dominates rather than other kinds of psychological or social purposes (Kirkpatrick, 2005).

This is perhaps the best explanation for the perplexing observation that religious traditions founded upon ethics of compassion, generosity, and love for others nevertheless can turn in a moment to coercion, intimidation, and violence toward those who are not members of the religious group. As Primo Levi observed in Auschwitz, "Compassion and brutality can coexist in the same individual and in the same moment, despite all logic" (Levi, 1988, p. 56). Those in religious outgroups—pagans, heathens, infidels, Jews, or gentiles—may not be recognized as full-blooded human beings. If not, there are no feelings of guilt if they are abused.

Social Hierarchy: "I Accept My Position within God's Order and Rule."

Within a single generation after its founding, nearly every religion has proposed a social order that claims to have originated by divine decree. Often, God or other supernatural beings are regarded as a powerful leader, the "alpha male," of the religious group. Exegeses of sacred scriptures provide rules, commandments, and other prescribed behaviors to which group members must submit in order to achieve status, prestige, honor, and respect. One gains closeness to God not through emotionally intimate interactions but through behavioral submission and obedience. Commonly, religious language reflects this psychology of social hierarchy, as in references to the kingdom of God or to God as ruler of all.

Galanter (1999, p. 4) has noted that religious cults are distinguished by the degree to which group behavioral norms influence group members' conduct and by imputing divine power to the cult leaders. The power of religion for prescribing a social hierarchy with attendant roles and responsibilities sets the stage for obedience to directives from group leaders, particularly if divinely attributed, even though they may conflict with a group member's spontaneous feelings or moral reasoning. Buss (2005, pp. 344–345) has noted:

> Status, prestige, esteem, honor, respect, and rank are accorded differentially to individuals in all known groups. People devote tremendous effort to avoiding disrepute, dishonor, shame, humiliation, disgrace, and loss of face. Empirical evidence suggests that status and dominance hierarchies form quickly. ... If there were ever a reasonable candidate for a universal human motive, status striving would be at or near the top of the list.

Justified as obedience to God's rule and order, religious groups can neglect, exploit, or commit violence while preserving a sense of righteousness. When roles and responsibilities are perceived to be divinely prescribed, moral reasoning by individual persons is easily discounted.

Social Exchange and Reciprocal Altruism: "God Ensures That Life Will Be Fair and Just."

Most religions articulate ethical rules and norms that prescribe correct social behavior. In nearly every religion, there are moral precepts about reciprocal altruism, what constitutes fair social exchange, and how cheaters are to be caught and punished (Kirkpatrick, 2005, p. 257; Krebs, 2005). Lerner (1980) has proposed that an extrapolation of social contract thinking to the natural world may underlie a belief in a just world. People everywhere tend to believe that a moral quid pro quo is built into the normal workings of the natural world: People get their just desserts, the good are rewarded, and the wicked are punished. When bad things happen to good people, an unfortunate but common conclusion is that those who suffer must not have been good people after all. As Pargament (1997, p. 227) has noted, God is nearly always viewed as just, someone who does not punish or destroy without purpose but always for a good reason.

Social exchange and reciprocal altruism can set the stage for exploitation when an individual persists in roles or behaviors that entail abuse or neglect, because of an expectation that suffering in the present will be requited at some future time through cosmic justice. Perversely, it can transmute into scapegoating the unlucky when those who suffer misfortunes are further burdened by being labeled as moral transgressors.

The Scope of Sociobiology in Religious Life

Religion is perhaps so powerful because it activates many different sociobio- *VERY IMP.* logical systems simultaneously. Religion recruits not only attachment behaviors between an individual and his or her God but also social processes of peer affiliation with attendant alliances and coalitions; social hierarchy with dominance, submission, and status seeking; kin recognition with demarcation of an ingroup apart from outgroups; and expectations for a just social exchange that includes reciprocal altruism. These sociobiological systems shape a person's interpersonal and social worlds in ways that have aided *Homo sapiens* in prevailing as a species over the course of human evolution.

This line of thinking does not argue that religion itself was a product of evolution. Religion may be more like a hermit crab occupying old shells built by other creatures at earlier times. Presumably these sociobiological systems evolved initially for survival purposes unrelated to religion. Once available, however, they became recruited into use by the psychological and social agendas of religious life. Religion thus is more like music or marriage, using biologically evolved brain systems for social and psychological ends unrelated to the original processes that gave structure to the brain. Religion activates the full range of sociobiological systems, and so completely that one might have predicted its spontaneous appearance were it not already omnipresent in human life. What aids moral reasoning within religious life is mindfulness of the extent to which these sociobiological systems can dictate both the form and the content of religious behavior.

Spirituality and Well-Being of Individuals

Relief of personal suffering is a mission for religion that appears to have originated independently from its ties to sociobiology. Between 800 B.C.E. and 700 C.E., charismatic religious leaders emerged who helped transform religion from its archaic tribal orientations to focus on the moral self-consciousness of individuals (Barnes, 2000, 2003; Armstrong, 1993). These religious leaders sought to discriminate institutionalized religious practices from an individual's personal religious experience, with the latter emphasizing beliefs, practices, and communal ways of living that alleviated suffering of individuals. They moved religion's field of interest from away from welfare of the group to the interior lives of individuals. The fruit of their labors was the emergence of personal spirituality as a form of religion within which the lived experience of an individual person is given priority.

Personal spirituality emerged at different locations worldwide within a narrow span of time. Lao Tzu, a succession of Hebrew prophets, Jesus Christ, the Buddha, and Mohammed were among the leaders who presented new religious beliefs and practices and reinterpreted older ones. Each of these innovative religious movements has continued until the present as a source of inspiration for individuals committed to personal tranquility and compassion toward others. Motivated more by moral reflection than sociobiological agendas, these religious reformations have been commonly referred to as spiritualities. These spiritualities were sometimes coopted and reinstitutionalized by later generations of their followers, who kept the names but made their contents concrete and formulaic. Yet each has also stood the test of time by continuing to nurture the moral reasoning, self-reflection, and personal growth for many who adhere to them.

The most intense religious ferment occurred during the 800–200 B.C.E. period, termed the Axial Age by Karl Jaspers (1953). In A History of God, Karen Armstrong (1993, p. 391) characterized the religious transformations of this historical era as follows:

Compassion was a characteristic of most of the ideologies that were created during the Axial Age. The compassionate ideal even impelled Buddhists to make a major change in their religious orientation when they introduced ✓devotion (*bhakti*) to the Buddha and *bodhisattvas*. The prophets insisted that cult and worship were useless unless society as a whole adopted a more just and compassionate ethos. These insights were developed by Jesus, Paul and the Rabbis, who all shared the same Jewish ideals and suggested major changes in Judaism to implement them. The Koran made the creation of a compassionate and just society the essence of the reformed religion of al-Lah. Compassion is a particularly difficult virtue. It demands that we go beyond the limitations of our egotism, insecurity and inherited prejudice.

Spiritualities associated with Taoism, Judaism, Christianity, Islam, Buddhism, and other traditions shared notable themes. These themes have been central as well for the work of more recent spiritual leaders, from Mahatma Gandhi to Mother Theresa and Martin Luther King[1]:

1. *Whole-person relatedness.* Spiritualities give primacy to "whole-person to whole-person" relatedness, which means opening oneself and responding fully to the other as a person. Interest in understanding the other's experience, despite acknowledged differences, is characteristic. Distinctions about social status, class, ethnicity, gender, or other such social categories are put aside. Whole-person relatedness fosters dialogue in which back-and-forth speaking, listening, and reflecting occur. Differing perspectives can be articulated, each considered respectfully, side by side. This relatedness has been described by Martin Buber as "I–Thou" rather than "I–It" relations (Buber, 1958). Emmanuel Levinas characterized such rapport between individuals as a "face-to-face relationship" that in its ethics seeks a good beyond being (Levinas, 1961). Anthropologist Victor Turner (1969, 1974, 1982) described it in terms of a social process of "communitas," evident during ritual observances when distinctions around social hierarchy and boundaries disappear, a powerful awareness of bonds that connect people takes hold, with "men in their wholeness wholly attending" (Turner, 1969, p 128).

2. *Commitment to an ethic of compassion.* Even the most inward focused of spiritualities ends consistently in an ethics of compassion toward other human beings. This compassion means that one responds to the suffering of any other person with understanding, caring, and efforts to heal or protect, without regard to social status. In some spiritualities, this ethic of compassion is extended to all living creatures (Armstrong, 1993).

---

[1] These themes of spirituality have been discussed in greater depth in *Encountering the Sacred in Psychotherapy* (Griffith & Griffith, 2002, Ch. 1).

3. *Compassionate care for self.* Compassion for others is reflexively extended to self as well by most spiritualities. This compassion shared with others is distinguished from narcissistic care for self that is built upon indifference toward others. Compassionate care for self provides containment for personal woundedness, which interrupts cycles of revenge and retaliation.

4. *Emotional postures of resilience.* Spiritualities typically generate coherency, hope, purpose, gratitude, joy, and other existential postures that confer personal resilience in the face of threat, uncertainty, and suffering (Griffith & Griffith, 2002).

5. *Encounters with the sacred as personal, evocative experiences that stimulate reflection, moral reasoning, and creativity.* In a generic sense, the sacred is regarded as the realm of human encounters with suprahuman agency, such as the actions of supernatural forces, gods, spirits, or transcendental reality. Within spirituality, such experiences lead to personal reflection rather than to efforts to use the power of the sacred to control other individuals through magic, as in primitive religions, or to rule societies or fight enemies, as has often happened in classical religions.

6. Prioritizing the well-being of individual persons, whether self or others, over the needs of religious groups. Spirituality is person-centered religion.

These six themes of spiritualities are only some of those of concern to theologians and psychologists of religion. However, they do catch a great deal of what quickly becomes problematic about religion in their absence. Attention to these six themes helps monitor what is missing when religious life becomes defined solely by its sociobiological agendas.

Relationally, these themes span the scope of human relatedness with self, with others, and with the divine. Relatedness exists both interpersonally and intrapersonally, both between people and within the self. Whole-person relatedness and a personal ethic of compassion are mainly directed toward interpersonal domains. Encounters with the sacred, compassionate care of self, and generation of existential postures of resilience largely operate intrapersonally. Prioritizing the well-being of an individual over group concerns is an ethical commitment that spans both interpersonal and intrapersonal spheres of relations. The message of spirituality is that religion is about connection, whether with self, other people, or the divine. As Prince Myshkin, Dostoevsky's exemplar of spirituality, put it, "It's just laziness that makes people classify themselves according to appearances, and fail to find anything in common" (Dostoevsky, 1869/2004, p. 25).

These themes of spirituality also underscore how religion is about social cognition. Sociobiological religion, but not personal spirituality, is formed by perceptual distinctions that are regulated by the different sociobiological systems. Personal spirituality, on the other hand, is mainly formed by perceptual distinctions involving attunement to emotional states of individuals.

Spirituality Provides What Sociobiology and Biological Evolution Failed to Provide

Spirituality can be regarded as a person-centered corrective for what biological evolution and sociobiology failed to provide. Personal spirituality is religion for the person. It adds to religious life a capacity for managing suffering inherent in an individual's lived experience, overriding sorrow and demoralization with hope, purpose, communion, and joy, helping people desire to live because life's pains can be made bearable. Its value was captured in the life and words of Albert Camus, a man who was pointedly nonreligious: "In the depth of winter I finally learned that within me there lay an invincible summer" (Klempner, 2006, p. 19).

Well-being of individual persons is not of particular consequence for biological evolution. The suffering of any particular person rarely, if ever, could imperil the species. To the contrary, early disappearance of weak individuals by death or failure to reproduce could strengthen the gene pool. Personal spirituality motivates compassion and care of the weak even when this does not make good evolutionary sense.

By contrast, sociobiological systems evolved because they were effective in promoting survival for the human species as a whole. Sociobiological systems are each teleological, imbued with specific purposes and ends within a social world: a mothering attachment; peer relationships; a social structure with roles, responsibilities, and leadership that ensures work gets done and enemies are kept at bay. The sociobiological systems share a general behavioral program with other mammals. To the extent that a successful group accrues benefits for individuals within it, sociobiological systems can enhance the well-being and enjoyment of its individual members, but this is a by-product when it happens, not a primary aim. Like a winning political party or an army dividing the spoils of victory, there are advantages to serving on the winning side. However, this kind of "good" does not necessarily enrich or enliven an individual's existence.

The behavioral programs of personal spirituality often go far afield from evolutionary aims dictated by inclusive fitness. Each sociobiological system has its primary task to accomplish, and personal spirituality serves none of them well. As discussed in the next chapter, compassion, an important theme in personal spirituality, was built upon an evolutionary platform of pain systems for detecting physical threats and avoiding them. In the emotional ethics of spirituality, however, compassion initiates movements that differ in direction from the design directives of a physical pain system, sometimes even moving toward, instead of away from, a source of pain when care of another person requires it.

Placing spirituality on a time line within human history risks implying that personal spirituality is "mature" religion, while sociobiological religion is "primitive." Indeed, a recent trend in North American and European culture has been to demarcate sharply the distinctions between religion and spirituality, regarding spirituality as personal, self-realizing, and creative but religion as institutional, rule driven, and stultifying (Hood et al., 2009). Human life seems more complex than that (Zinnbauer & Pargament, 2005).

Personal spirituality and sociobiological religion may differ in fundamental ways, but the differences simply mean that they are useful for different ends. Except under pathological conditions, personal spirituality and sociobiological religion typically operate in harmony. There are rare Dag Hammarskjolds who live lives of profound personal spirituality absent any formal religious structure, but they are exceptional (Hammarskjold, 1964). As Pargament (2007) has noted, empirical studies of religiousness find that the vast majority of religious people access spirituality through their formal religious practices. For example, the observance of Seder is a ritual that lies at the heart of Judaism as an organized religious tradition. For many, it also is the heart of personal spirituality, as an encounter with the sacred, a source of purpose, and a point of communion with fellow worshippers, past, present, and future. Other religious traditions likewise provide specific methods and means that are intended as paths to spirituality by utilizing their beliefs, spiritual practices, sacred stories, rituals, and communities (Griffith & Griffith, 2002).

Leaders who have introduced spirituality into their societies, whether the prophet Isaiah or St. Francis of Assisi, usually have been astute in navigating their sociobiological religious contexts, enough at least for delivering their messages. Some, like Mahatma Gandhi, have been politically savvy and utilized their knowledge of religious sociobiology to mobilize populations for effective action. By contrast, Prince Myshkin in *The Idiot* was seemingly unable to take stock of the hierarchies, boundaries, and role expectations guiding others around him. The power of his person-focused empathy and compassion opened relationships even with those who wanted to dismiss him. Nevertheless, his acts of compassion, blind to their sociobiological contexts, ended tragically for those he tried to help and left the prince in an insane asylum (Dostoevsky, 1869/2004). Spirituality may take a leading role in religious life, yet still needs adequate input from a sociobiological perspective for its missions to be realized.

Awareness of sociobiology clarifies that religion is about more than spirituality when people speak prayers, observe rituals, and attend churches, temples, and mosques. Religion is validly also about friendships, finding community, teaming with others to pursue common goods, and knowing "to whom I belong," aims other than those of personal spirituality.

Personal spirituality can be regarded as a reformation of religion to accommodate emergence of a moral individual self. It is one possible outcome of religious life. Personal spirituality emerged out of a human history of religious sociobiology, and the two cannot be separated as if they bore no kinship. Personal spirituality often needs the structure of organized religion. It can be effervescent, dissipating over time without some support from traditional religious beliefs, practices, or community life. Personal spirituality and sociobiological religion are the muscle and bone of religious life, inseparable in any religion that is vibrant. Both the differentness and kinship between them are keys to understanding how religion so powerfully effects healing in some contexts and harm in others.

Personal Spirituality and Sociobiological Religion Sometimes Sharply Diverge

As a general rule, religion risks destructive consequences for individuals when any of six themes of personal spirituality discussed previously is constricted or absent, such that religiousness becomes defined solely by its sociobiology. Sociobiological religion is constituted by its responses to normative specifications from social systems. Spirituality, like art, is constituted by creative expressions of individual sensibilities. When religious life ceases to function as a medium for individual expression, risks enter for potential harm to persons.

Personal spirituality and sociobiological religion can diverge at points of vulnerability when their primary aims fail to dovetail. There is a built-in tension. Many of the gravest abuses of religion involve violence toward "the stranger" who is outside the religious group. Racism or tribalism is a natural consequence when kin recognition and peer affiliation obscure commitment to whole-person relatedness with those in outgroups. Members of religious groups are themselves at risk when submission to role and authority negates a compassionate relatedness toward self, as vividly recounted in Karen Armstrong's (2004) *The Spiral Staircase*. Powerfully experienced encounters with the sacred, common within personal spirituality, often lead individuals into idiosyncratic paths at odds with the religious behaviors prescribed by ecclesiastical authorities.

Polish foreign correspondent Ryszard Kapuscinski (2008, p. 36) described well this human conundrum as he reflected on the violence he witnessed firsthand in Africa, Asia, and Central America: "Man when he is alone is usually more 'human' than when he is a member of a crowd, an excited mass. Individually, we are wiser and better, less inscrutable. Becoming part of a group can change the same quiet, friendly individual into a devil." Sociobiological religion is a source of "crowd-ness" in religious life, and personal spirituality a source of its "alone-ness."

The clinical case illustrations in these chapters largely focus on interventions that draw upon the themes of personal spirituality—whole-person relatedness, an ethic of compassion, personal encounters with the sacred, mobilization of existential of resilience, and prioritizing of person over group—to restore a voice of spirituality within religiously informed decision making by medical and psychiatric patients.

Making Sense of Harmful Religious Behaviors

A sociobiological perspective helps a clinician to grasp perplexing cognitive and emotional perspectives that might not be otherwise intuited when patients have strong religious, or ideological, identities. Chapter 6 extends this sociobiological discussion to explain how patients belonging to tightly cohesive religious or ideological groups can operate with dual selves—a public sociobiological self and a private personal self—each with its own circumscribed awareness, sensibilities, values, and commitments. Only the sociobiological self may be revealed in a clinical encounter. This sociobiological self is particularly sensitive to a clinician's actions when they touch on attachment, peer affiliation, kin recognition, social hierarchy, and social exchange relations. Such an understanding can provide critical guidance when interacting with patients and planning therapeutic interventions.

Assessing whether themes of personal spirituality are present or absent in a patient's religiousness is key to gauging risks of potential harm. This assessment walks a fine line between intervening for justifiable clinical and ethical reasons and respecting a patient's right to practice a religious faith however he or she chooses. Destructive uses of religion are sometimes so explicit as to require little discussion, as with religious justifications for racist acts or domestic violence. An ethical or legal obligation to impose control exists when there is imminent risk of harm, as with threats of suicide or violence. More often, harmful effects are less extreme and more subtle. Then it is best to try to engage the patient as a collaborator in discerning the real-life effects that his or her religious behaviors have on self or others.

The clinician's role is one of consultant to a patient's moral decision making. The clinician's aim is to aid a patient in noticing moral impulses from one's personal spirituality that can help inform ethical discernments. An awareness of the themes of spirituality that religion ought to bring forth in a person's life guides assessment. Specific questions can help discern whether religious practices support relational dimensions of spirituality. Examples of such questions include:

- ✦ Does the patient's attachment style with his or her God promote security or insecurity?
- ✦ Do religious encounters with the sacred evoke fear or aggression, or do they stimulate reflection and creativity?
- ✦ Are interactions with others in the patient's religious group dialogical or monological in character? That is, can a person, regardless of role or status, expect to be able to speak, to be heard and understood, and to have one's perspective taken seriously within the group? How is the least powerful person treated?
- ✦ What kind of person would feel embarrassed or ill at ease in this gathering?
- ✦ How are people in outgroups regarded? In practice, are they respected and valued as full human beings?
- ✦ Is ethical decision making guided by whether a person is first identified as an ingroup or outgroup member?

The practice of a religious faith also should support such existential postures as coherence, hope, communion, agency, purpose, commitment, and gratitude. These existential postures are essential for care of self in the face of adversity. A red flag of concern is raised when the fruits of religious practices are not these, but rather confusion, despair, isolation, helplessness, meaninglessness, detachment, or resentment (Griffith & Griffith, 2002). A clinician can inquire how well these existential postures are supported by a patient's attachment style with God, peer affiliation within the religious group, relatedness with those in outgroups, and ethical practices grounded in just expectations for social exchange.

2

What Neurobiology Explains
about Destructive Uses of Religion

THE WORKINGS OF SOCIOBIOLOGICAL RELIGION AND PERSONAL
spirituality extend beyond the interpersonal sphere into the physical brains of
involved individuals. Religious experience is embodied. Religious experience
shapes and is shaped by the physiological state of the nervous system. The
physical structure of the human brain in part accounts for a tenuous coexistence between sociobiological religion and personal spirituality.

Neurobiology is the scientific study of the nervous system and how its
cells are organized into functional units that process information and initiate behaviors (Shepard, 1994). Human neurobiology includes research studies
utilizing functional brain imaging that permits visualization of specific brain
behavioral circuits as they influence or are influenced by psychological states
and social behaviors. Such research is providing a window into interactions
that may occur between brain physiology and the religious lives of individuals.

Why Neurobiology Matters

Every religion presents methods for optimizing religious experience by altering the state of the brain. Eyes are closed during prayers to eliminate brain
activation by visual stimuli. Meditation and chanting are used to lower brain

arousal. Fasting, dietary rituals, and ingesting sacred foods attempt to alter the brain by regulating its nutritional supplies. Sweat lodges overheat the brain. Mescaline or other psychoactive substances are used to reconfigure the brain's perceptual systems in sacred rituals (Albaugh & Anderson, 1974). The rituals and practices of our mainstream Western religions—the Eucharist, the Shab-bat, chanting monks, muezzins beckoning to evening prayers—are each in part an attempt to bring mind and body into unspoken harmony (Griffith & Griffith, 2002).

Effects are also causal in the opposite direction. Religious experiences can produce powerful shifts in activation of certain brain circuits, with important consequences for both religious and nonreligious sectors of life. Religion can help activate or deactivate brain systems for empathy and compassion. It also can facilitate or inhibit brain systems for reflective thought, self-awareness, and regulation of emotional states. In moments of religious zeal, religion can amplify emotional states beyond the range within which they can be con-trolled by internal thought or will. As a loose analogy, we can think of reli-gion in these roles as we might regard a mind-altering drug. These effects matter in daily life with family, friends, and acquaintances as well as with strangers who live beyond the city walls.

There are only rare occasions when aberrant brain activity produces symptoms, such as delusional thinking, that drive religion directly toward destructive ends. Rather, neurobiology's participation in destructive expres-sions of religion is usually a negative, subtractive role. Harmful religious behaviors are often associated with neurobiological deactivation of brain systems that support interpersonal relatedness, empathy, compassion, moral reflection, and dialogue.

Traumatic stress or threats to group security can trigger a global deacti-vation of brain systems necessary for processes of personal spirituality. Ter-ror, horror, helplessness, and humiliation are common precipitants for the sequenced shutting down of brain capacities for empathy, compassion, reflec-tion, or dialogue. The human body is evolutionarily programmed to further survival. The body of a starving man automatically burns sugar stores before fat, fat before muscle, and muscle before vital organs. The metabolic rate of a starving body drops to levels that sustain the functioning of only those body systems essential for survival. In an analogous manner, the brain of a per-son who feels threatened or insecure begins shutting down neural networks that are not essential to personal or group survival. The major sociobiological systems—attachment, kin recognition, peer affiliation—guide this triaging of brain resources. Relatedness with strangers is often the first set of functions to disappear. Religious experiences that evoke fear, uncertainty, or insecurity

can themselves send the brain into survival mode, sometimes with consequent loss of relatedness toward those outside one's own group.

Relatedness toward others also can be switched off during routine daily
life despite normal levels of arousal. The major sociobiological systems support
the social structures of group life in families, organizations, communities, and
societies. They perform this function by organizing people within social roles
and categories, not their individuality. Empathy for specific persons or groups
can be switched off if social dominance or kin recognition systems are so cued
in order to reestablish social hierarchy. Understanding these processes starts
with the neurobiology of empathy.

The Pain Matrix and Empathy

All animals have evolved pain circuits within their nervous systems that
detect threats to survival and initiate evasive and avoidant movements. The
core pain systems of most animals consist of sensory receptors placed throughout the body to detect damage to tissues. These receptors send neural impulses
over nerves to the spinal cord, which transmits the information to the thalamus, a sensory way station atop the brainstem. The thalamus, in turn, activates regions of the cerebral cortex to program muscle movements for leaving
the vicinity of the painful stimulus. Circuits at the level of brainstem and
spinal cord operate automatically and unconsciously in their reflex responses.
Those within the cerebral cortex also involve conscious awareness and volitional responses. (See Figure 2.1.)

In human beings, a "pain matrix" has evolved that has multiple levels of
pain perception, analgesic, and motor responses. It detects pain as a danger
signal and initiates self-protective actions. The pain matrix has two separate
divisions for perceiving different dimensions of pain. One gauges the intensity
of suffering, while the other merely maps the location of the pain and registers its sensory characteristics, whether burning, cutting, tearing, or electric
shock-like (Albanese, Duerden, Rainville, & Duncans, 2007). At the highest
level of the cerebral cortex, the anterior cingulate gyrus and insula have the
major roles of monitoring the intensity of suffering, while the sensory cortex
of the parietal lobe has the major role of monitoring sensory qualities of pain.
In addition to structures for perceiving pain, the pain matrix also includes
components such as the motor cortex and cerebellum that stage movements
away from the painful stimulus (Jackson, Rainville, & Decety, 2006; Decety
& Grezes, 2006).

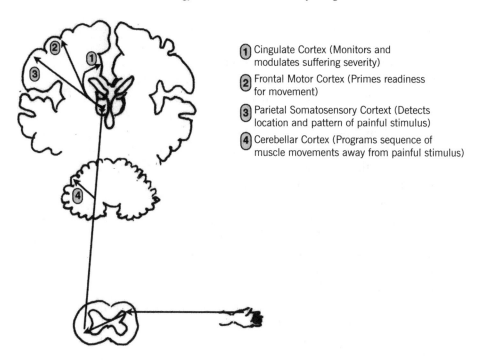

① Cingulate Cortex (Monitors and modulates suffering severity)

② Frontal Motor Cortex (Primes readiness for movement)

③ Parietal Somatosensory Cortext (Detects location and pattern of painful stimulus)

④ Cerebellar Cortex (Programs sequence of muscle movements away from painful stimulus)

FIGURE 2.1. The pain matrix. The pain matrix integrates sensory pain perception with motor responses to avoid painful stimuli and analgesic mechanisms to attenuate unavoidable suffering. Brainstem and spinal cord circuits operate automatically outside conscious awareness, while those within the cerebral cortex also involve conscious awareness and volitional responses. In mammals, the pain matrix also responds to threats to vital relationships (attachment system). In humans, it also responds vicariously to pain experienced by another person (empathy).

The pain matrix is intimately connected to analgesia systems for shutting down the felt perception of pain. Analgesia systems either screen out pain sensations entirely or limit their impact. They include perspective taking, hypnosis, and the placebo response as cognitive controls over pain, together with the brain's internal opiate (enkephalin) system and sensory-gating mechanisms in the spinal cord that enable counterstimulation measures, such as scratching or rubbing, to reduce pain.

The processing of incoming information as it rises through the brain's sensory systems toward the cerebral cortex is termed "bottom-up processing." Activation of the pain matrix by physical, emotional, or vicarious perceptions of painful experiences are examples of bottom-up processing. Analgesia systems and other brain circuits that modify the intensity or alter the quality of incoming information provide "top-down processing." Top-down processing, in which incoming pain sensations are buffered or eliminated, plays an important role in helping people adapt to their environment. For example, Tucker, Luu, and Derryberry (2005) have noted how young mammals separated from their mother emit sounds of distress. Small doses of opiates stop the distress vocalizations and cause the animals' searching for their mother to cease, an example of pharmacological top-down regulation. Another example is hypnosis that uses the top-down regulation by the prefrontal cortex to suppress activation of the anterior cingulate gyrus by pain sensations.

The splitting of somatosensory pain perception from affective pain perception is part of the structural design of the nervous system at every level from the periphery to the cerebral cortex. This anatomic division enables behavioral coping responses to pain to keep their focus without undue distraction from the suffering element. Behavioral responses to escape the painful stimulus proceed under guidance of parietal somatosensory cortex, which monitors location and qualities of sensations. The affective processing of insula and cingulate cortex meanwhile can be dampened by top-down regulation from prefrontal and dorsal cingulate cortex systems.

This modular organization of the pain matrix—a reconnaissance module to lock onto location and qualities of pain sensations (somatosensory cortex), an affective module to gauge the misery index of the pain (insula, anterior cingulate cortex), a motor response module for physical escape from the painful stimulus (frontal motor cortex, cerebellum)—is a physical fact of the nervous system that also structures the most intimate experiences of living in the world. Humans are designed with a capacity to keep a cognitive focus on sensory details of a physical world and what is happening in it, while modulating the intensity of the felt experience of it.

Although the pain matrix originally evolved to sound alarm about physical injury, elaboration of the mammalian attachment system redirected its responses to emotional pains as well (Tucker et al., 2005). Cries of distress from an infant separated from its mother activate the pain matrix just as much as physical pain. The purview of the pain matrix thus has been extended to include not only tissue damage but also the threatened loss of a vital relationship (Tucker et al., 2005).

The pain matrix also provides a neural infrastructure for empathy. Vicarious experiencing of another person's pain activates the same structures within the brain as does pain in one's physical body (Jackson et al., 2006). Over the course of evolution, the original function of the pain matrix for managing physical pain was doubly co-opted, first by adapting it to respond to emotional

as well as to physical pain and then by adapting it further to respond to pain
in other people. Acts of compassion became vehicles for regulating pain that
is vicariously experienced.

Mirror Neurons and Compassion

Adapting the pain matrix for other-directed empathy required the biological
evolution of a mirror neuron system. When mirror neurons were introduced
into the brains of mammals, the sensing of one's own physical and emotional
pain began to include sensing that of others as well. This awareness of the
other's experience became a first step toward compassion.

Discovery of mirror neurons in the frontal lobe of the brain in the 1980s
captivated the imaginations of neuroscientists (Rizolatti & Craighero, 2004).
Neuroscientists were accustomed to thinking about the individual person as
the unit for biological investigation. Pain sensations from sensory receptors in
the skin and other peripheral body parts were understood to travel through
pain fibers to the brain where they would activate nociceptive circuits. Likewise, touch sensations would travel to the brain and activate somesthetic
circuits and so forth for visual, auditory, taste, and smell sensations. In the
cerebral cortex, executive systems such as the prefrontal cortex would then
integrate all this information in complex three-dimensional, time-extensive,
cognitive and emotional pictures of the person's world. Mirror neurons, however, were discovered to activate not only in response to events in a person's
own life but also when events were happening to other people. Circuits for
facial movements activated while watching movements of another person's
face. Pain matrix activation occurred not only when one's own body was
injured but also when another person's pain was being witnessed.

The existence of mirror neurons suggested that people use simulation
to understand other people (Oberman & Ramachandran, 2007). That is, an
individual perceiving another person in a certain situation automatically and
unconsciously re-creates that perception within the observer's own motor,
cognitive, or emotional neural networks, in essence running an "offline simulation." This offline simulation gives one access to an embodied understanding of the other person's actions or expressions. We thus have a way to feel
the thoughts, behaviors, or emotions of another person within our own bodies
(Ruby & Decety, 2004).

Mirror neurons were discovered to be particularly concentrated in two
major locations: the cortex of the inferior frontal lobe and superior sulcus of
the temporal lobe. These neurons respond to actions of others. Inform;

gathered by these mirror neurons is then dispersed frontward and backward, frontward to the executive control systems of the prefrontal cortex and backward to the parietal cortex. This frontal–temporal–parietal network constitutes the core of a mirror neuron system for understanding other people and their behaviors.

Interestingly, a region of parietal cortex receiving mirror neuron information has also been known as Wernicke's area in the left, dominant hemisphere. For 100 years, Wernicke's area has been known to be responsible for decoding symbolic communication and the understanding of language. Similarly, a region of the inferior frontal lobe containing mirror neurons has also been known as Broca's area, a brain region responsible for using language to compose the motor programs of speech and writing. The brain system for understanding the experiences of others thus overlays the brain systems for understanding language and for communicating with others. This has suggested to some that spoken language may have evolved from physical gestures. Their proximity underscores the close relationship between dialogue and empathic attunement in relationships, to which such existentialist philosophers as Martin Heidegger, Martin Buber, and Emmanuel Levinas have attributed central importance (Buber, 1958; Heidegger, 1962, 1971; Levinas, 1961, 1981/1997; see Figure 2.2).

Discovery of mirror neurons led to the "theory-of-mind" hypothesis, or mentalization. The theory-of-mind hypothesis proposed that a person performs internal simulations of perceived actions and then uses that awareness of one's own actions and intentions to infer what the other must be thinking,

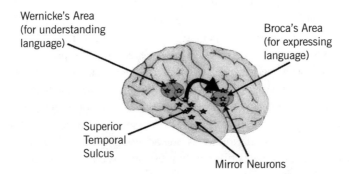

FIGURE 2.2. Mirror neuron and language systems. The mirror neuron system largely overlays Wernicke's area for language perception and Broca's area for language expression, providing an anatomic foundation for the close relationship between dialogue and emotional intimacy.

feeling, and intending. Monitoring one's own internal state is thus a prerequisite for predicting the behavior of others (Ruby & Decety, 2004). Mentalization provided a solution for the old philosophical problem of solipsism: How is it that we can know with confidence what is in the mind of another person? We know it because the other's experience becomes physically reconstructed within our own nervous systems. Within our own being, we feel the experience of the other. ᴏʀ ɴᴏᴛ — theris the puzzle · cf p 44

Self and Other Are Together—and Apart— within the Brain

Permitting one's own pain matrix to be activated by another's distress makes possible empathy and compassion. However, it also introduces potential confusion between self and other. Whose pain is it when one's pain matrix activates? This is, of course, a problem in real life when two people are closely and empathically joined. A mother feels her children's pains and lovers feel each other's pains to the point that whose pain it is becomes unclear. Such confusion is a core deficit in psychotic mental disorders, such as schizophrenia, when one's own thoughts may be heard from the outside-like voices talking and communications from others are felt coming from inside one's own being. Most people, however, are able to keep track of what are first-person experiences and what are vicarious, third-person experiences.

The brain is structurally organized in at least two ways to enable experiences of self to be distinguished from experiences of others. This brain organization involves the anterior cingulate cortex and insula, which are the final destinations for pain matrix information regarding suffering, and the sensory cortex of the parietal lobe, which is the final destination for pain matrix information regarding sensory qualities of pain.

First, sensory information about others is stored in close proximity, but not quite identical in location to information about others. Sensory perceptions about physical pain in a person's own body are mapped into the bottom regions of the insula and anterior cingulate cortex, while perceptions of pain in other persons are stored more to the top and front of each (Decety & Grezes, 2006).

Second, the parietal regions of the two cerebral hemispheres work in concert to distinguish experiences of self from experiences of another person. The right side of the brain is largely organized as a default system to guarantee personal survival. It prioritizes emotional awareness of self as a physical body. Right-hemisphere brain systems favor rapid responses to environmental events that are based on pattern perception and emotions, not detailed analyses and reflective thought. The left side of the brain is better organized for relatedness to a world outside oneself, including relationships with other people. The left hemisphere provides language, complex logical analyses, and mentalization of the minds of others. By comparing their patterns of activation, the parietal regions of the two hemispheres can keep track of what is self and what is other, what is inside and what is outside of self.

These distinctions also enable a sense of agency, which is an awareness of whether actions are initiated by self or by other and "who did what to whom" (Decety & Grezes, 2006; Lamm et al., 2007). Unless disrupted by stress, the brain is usually able to distinguish first-person from third-person experiences.

Mentalization and Empathy Are Not the Same

Mentalization provides the first bridge from one's own experiential world to that of another. Through mentalization, a person can discern how behaviors of other people are due to their intentional mental states. One can surmise, "If I were in that situation, what would I be noticing? What options might I consider in dealing with it?" Mentalizing is the capacity to imagine the mental state of another person in a manner that makes psychological sense out of that person's feelings, thoughts, and actions. Sometimes this is done as a deliberate, thoughtful process. However, most mentalizing occurs at a preconscious level (Bateman & Fonagy, 2006). This ability to put oneself in the place of another person, and to imagine what the other might be thinking, appears to have been a critical evolutionary advantage that *Homo sapiens* held over other early hominids (Mithen, 1996, p. 50).

Although mentalization infers the thinking of another person, it stops short of feeling the other person's experience as if it were one's own. Mentalizing regards emotional expressions of the other as one more stream of information. However, this does not necessarily carry over to feeling those emotions firsthand. A leading theory of psychopathy proposes that psychopaths are skilled mentalizers but incapable of empathy because of flawed limbic circuits (Abbott, 2001, 2007; Kiehl, 2006). Psychopaths can make psychologically sophisticated observations about the behaviors of other people, appraise their motivations and habits, and use this knowledge to manipulate and prey upon them, all the while never feeling the other's pain. Neurobiologically, psychopaths lack an integration of a third-person, cognitive perspective with a first-person, emotional perspective of the other's experience.

Empathy relies upon accurate appraisal of the emotional perspective of the other. The region of the prefrontal cortex located just behind the eyes—the medial prefrontal cortex—serves a key role in emotional perspective taking (Hynes, Baird, & Grafton, 2006). When observing another person, the medial prefrontal cortex constructs an "emotional image" of the experience of the other by bringing together information from a variety of sources:

+ The amygdala ascertains the emotional valence of incoming information.
+ Information from mirror neurons in the superior temporal sulcus registers the other person's expressions of thoughts, feelings, and intentions.
+ Temporal lobe cortex retrieves stored information of memories that might aid interpretation.

The medial prefrontal cortex links these different streams of cognitive information with emotional arousal appropriate in kind and intensity, thereby producing an emotional perspective about the experience of the other. A person can then use this emotional perspective to guide how he or she acts toward the other.

Among all the brain regions, the more dorsomedial prefrontal cortex (Brodmann's areas 8, 9, 10) is particularly critical for the attribution of mental states to other people (Farrow et al., 2001; Jackson et al., 2006). Closely adjacent ventral medial prefrontal areas (Brodmann's areas 11 and 25) serve specific key roles in emotional perspective taking (Hynes et al., 2006; Seitz, Nichel, & Azari, 2006; see Figure 2.3).

Empathy for Strangers Occurs Naturally

What limited empirical research that has been conducted suggests that people naturally experience empathy for others. Milamaaria et al. (2007) found that humans naturally experienced empathy for strangers in pain, at least under scientific laboratory conditions. Their conclusion, however, stands in puzzling contrast to the conclusions of Primo Levi from Auschwitz: "Many people—many nations—can find themselves holding, more or less wittingly, that 'every stranger is an enemy'" (1958/1996, p. 9). What might account for the difference between a laboratory scientific experiment and a Nazi death camp as a real-world social experiment? The answer must lie not within the structure of

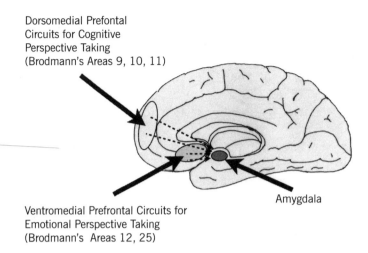

Dorsomedial Prefontal
Circuits for Cognitive
Perspective Taking
(Brodmann's Areas 9, 10, 11)

Amygdala

Ventromedial Prefrontal Circuits for
Emotional Perspective Taking
(Brodmann's Areas 12, 25)

FIGURE 2.3. Cognitive and emotional perspective-taking circuits of the medial prefrontal cortex. Cognitive perspective taking (grasping how another person perceives and reasons) is centered in "theory-of-mind" circuits of the dorsomedial prefrontal cortex. Emotional perspective taking (grasping the felt experience of another person) relies particularly upon the ventromedial prefrontal cortex. Both regions provide top-down regulation of threat and avoidance responses of the amygdala. In its fullest sense, empathy involves both cognitive and emotional perspective taking.

the nervous system but in the differing social contexts and the influences of society, which the controlled conditions of a laboratory carefully shield out. Under real-life conditions, social factors dictate how brain circuits that support empathic attunement are activated or deactivated.

Empathy within the brain has three major components: (1) experiencing the emotional perspective of the other; (2) generating an affective response toward the other; (3) monitoring the origin of feelings, whether arising from self or from the other (Lamm et al., 2007; Tucker et al., 2005). Empathy is aborted when neural circuits enabling any of these three components fail to operate. There are neuropsychiatric disorders, for example, in which the brain circuits associated with empathy are damaged or dysfunctional. Patients with autism are largely unable to experience empathy because their mirror neuron system fails to activate (Dapretto et al., 2006). Patients with frontotemporal dementias or strokes lose a capacity for empathy because of a damaged medial prefrontal cortex (Shamay-Tsoory, Tomer, Berger, Goldsher, & Aharon-Peretz, 2005). In psychopathy and in callous-unemotional youth with conduct disor-

ders, the amygdala and associated limbic circuits appear damaged and unable
to generate emotional responses (Dolan, 2008)

A person with a normal brain may nevertheless fail to show empathy
when social cues disrupt activation of the empathy system. Moreover, social
cues sometimes even prompt the prefrontal cortex to shift activation away
from the pain matrix toward the reward systems of the striatum instead. For
example, detection of a competitor or a cheater in a social encounter switches
activation from anterior cingulate cortex (pain matrix) activation to striatum activation (reward system). A person feels satisfaction, not distress, when
competitors lose or cheaters are punished (de Quervain et al., 2004).

Two Different Kinds of "Otherness"

"Other" is a word that carries a puzzling ambiguity. On the one hand,
acknowledgement that others exist and movement toward relatedness with
others are sentinel signs of psychological development. On the other hand,
detection of an "other" in one's midst serves as a universal signal for alarm
and mobilization against potential threat. This dual face of otherness is
reflected in our clinical literatures. Some clinicians seeking reconciliation in
conflicted relationships adopt strategies that reduce hostility by dampening
perceptions of otherness in other people (Weingarten, 2003). Other clinicians adopt strategies that achieve similar ends by heightening awareness of
otherness (Meissner, 1987; Zinner, 2008). Perception of otherness as an opening to curiosity, intrigue, and awe, rather than threat and alarm, is a major
theme of this text.

This ambiguous character of otherness can be explained in part by its
potency for activating brain systems whose behavioral paths can diverge in
opposite directions. Perception of otherness can immediately set into play kin
recognition systems whose function is to distinguish ingroup members from
those of outgroups. If this prompts an alarm response, then peer affiliation
and social hierarchy systems are similarly mobilized in readiness to react to
threat. However, perception of otherness also can signal to mentalization and
empathy systems that there is someone of interest who needs to be known.
Cognitive and emotional perspective-taking circuits are brought into play
to grasp how this person thinks and feels and how relatedness might best
proceed. Despite their opposing teleologies, both systems for social cognition
are activated by perception of an "other," and the consequent direction that
behaviors take depends upon their relative influence in the balance.

Empathy Switches That Selectively Shut Down Relatedness toward Others

"Empathy switches" are top-down regulatory processes that extend or withdraw empathic responses to others, enabling empathy to be turned on or off selectively during daily life. Empathy switches can either shut off emotional awareness or redirect it, thereby facilitating avoidance behaviors such as fleeing from, or even attacking a person in pain.

Top-down regulatory systems of the medial and dorsal prefrontal cortex are prime candidates for service as empathy switches. The medial prefrontal cortex serves a variety of gating and information-filtering roles in its monitoring and controlling of information processing (Shimamura, 2000; Ochsner, 2007), particularly in regard to such social emotions as embarrassment, pride, shame, and guilt (Beer, 2007). The dorsal prefrontal cortex serves the major role in subjecting behavior to willful control guided by plans and ambitions rather than spontaneous feelings (Lieberman, 2007). These empathy switches represent an ongoing, dynamic interplay between theory-of-mind circuits and mirror neuron circuits. As social neuroscience researcher Christian Keysers (2009) put it, these theory-of-mind circuits are constantly "playing with the knobs" of empathy based upon appraisals of the other person's perspectives. A detailed understanding of these processes is still being elucidated. It is not yet clear how many different types of processes might operate as empathy switches and whether some may be implicit and automatic while others may be explicit and volitional. It has been not determined whether empathy switches operate by diverting mirror neuron information away from limbic or sensory cortex so that no emotions are generated or whether activation occurs in these areas that is subsequently suppressed. The relative extents to which these processes may represent learned social cognitions or automatic hardwired responses have not been clarified. Empathy switches may be created ephemerally within a virtual reality programmed to fit moment-to-moment appraisals of one's social circumstances, or they may operate within fixed neural circuits like rail yard switches that direct trains of emotional information down one track or another. A survey of current neuroscience research suggests that multiple kinds of processes are involved.

The need for empathy switches seems obvious. Selective withdrawal of empathy serves an important role in maintenance of social structure within groups. Parents withdraw empathy, albeit partially, when punishing children. Spouses sometimes withdraw empathy from each other in setting expectations for their relationship. Physicians, teachers, and police each withdraw empathy selectively at key junctures to aid them in the performance of their professional duties. Attorneys may withdraw empathy from everyone other than the sole client who has engaged their services. When social dominance or kin recognition come into place, empathy can be withdrawn for entire classes of people, as with stereotyping, discrimination, and stigmatization of certain groups. Again, as Primo Levi noted, "Compassion and brutality can coexist in the same individual and in the same moment, despite all logic" (1988, p. 56). Extension and withdrawal of empathy, moment to moment even within a single relationship, is part of the rhythm of normal social life. Just as our hands have 10 fingers with which to grasp objects, it perhaps should be not be surprising if our brains were designed with 10, or more, different types of implicit and explicit systems for extending and withdrawing empathy according to social contexts. These systems turn empathy into a tool for structuring our social worlds.

Generally, attention trumps emotion in information processing within the brain, and focus of attention directs where and how empathy can operate (Norris & Cacioppo, 2007). Awareness of another person's emotional distress can be moved on or off the stage of cognition depending on where focused attention is directed. Empathy switches shift a focus of attention or change a cognitive perspective so that automatic activation of empathy systems is disrupted (Lamm et al., 2007). Taking an alternative perspective can replace compassion with sadistic pleasure when watching another person suffer.

The anterior cingulate gyrus serves the major role of allocating focused attention, aligning it strategically according to long-term priorities (Eisenberger, Lieberman, & Williams, 2003). Empathy switches presumably influence how the anterior cingulate gyrus distributes the brain's attentional resources (Milamaaria et al., 2007). Singer et al. (2004) has used functional brain imaging to show how psychological measures of compassion are correlated with levels of activation of the anterior cingulate cortex.

The amygdala and the ventral sector of the anterior cingulate cortex are the major monitoring stations for noting when incoming information has emotional salience. Two regulatory systems—the dorsal sector of the anterior cingulate cortex and the lateral prefrontal cortex—provide top-down regulation that neutralizes negative affective states by inhibiting activation of the ventral anterior cingulate cortex (Ochsner, Bunge, Gross, & Gabrieli, 2002; Ochsner, 2007). This top-down regulation makes possible hypnosis, the placebo response, and the human capacity for expectations and beliefs to mitigate suffering. When cued to do so, these same regulatory systems can switch off the felt experience of others' pain as well.

Psychopathy does not provide a broad explanation for social violence and exploitation. No more than 1% of the population are psychopaths whose antisocial acts are due to damaged limbic circuitry (Abbott, 2007). Rather, empathy switches appear to operate in normal persons, sometimes enabling violence or neglect toward others by suppressing pain matrix activation when suffering is witnessed. The settings of empathy switches presumably are established by the prefrontal cortex in response to social cues from the sociobiological systems (Norris & Cacioppo, 2007).

Different Types of Empathy Switches

The major sociobiological systems hold enormous sway in their command of the brain's attentional resources. Recent social neuroscience experiments have used functional brain imaging to track activation of brain circuits during staged social interactions. These studies have pointed toward a number of putative empathy switches connected to specific sociobiological systems, including:

+ Threatened loss of a vital relationship (attachment).
+ Perception that the other is a stranger (kin recognition).
+ Assertion of dominance (social hierarchy).
+ Moral judgment that the other has violated a code of moral conduct (social exchange).

Each of these can dampen or terminate awareness of another's suffering by disrupting empathy.

Some empathy switches appear to be specifically fear avoidant. These include terror- and horror-driven responses with massive amygdala activation. In position emission tomography scan studies of patients with posttraumatic stress disorder, Rauch, Shin, and Phelps (2006) have demonstrated how reexperiencing traumatic memories powerfully activates amygdala threat systems, while deactivating brain regions involved with empathy, such as medial prefrontal cortex. Similarly, witnessing another person in pain in a naturalistic context can signal danger and promote a withdrawal response rather than empathy (Jackson et al., 2006; Lamm et al., 2007).

Other putative empathy switches produce an emotional detachment that secondarily short-circuits empathy. Detachment occurs when a perspective is adopted that a situation does not have emotional relevance for one's own life or when a person imagines an image of self unaffected by the situation (Lamm et al., 2007). Some mechanisms enabling detachment operate automatically outside of awareness as implicit systems. Other explicit mechanisms involve awareness and reflective thought (Lamm et al., 2007). Detachment and perspective taking can be used either to promote empathy or to negate it. They can support effectiveness of mindful, intended choices to divert one's attention empathically toward the perspective of the other (Jackson et al., 2006; Lamm et al., 2007) or nonempathically away from it (Gross, 2002).

A different group of empathy switches involve reward circuits that are activated when witnessing the suffering of someone else. Competition, for example, activates a prefrontal cortex and parietal cortex network that subserves executive planning, prioritizing, and strategizing functions as well as the insula that adjusts levels of autonomic arousal. This pattern differs from the one seen during cooperation (Decety, Jackson, Sommerville, Chaminade, & Meltzoft, 2004). As another example, the perception of fairness facilitates empathy, whereas unfairness or selfish behavior suppresses it (Singer et al., 2006; Hsu, Anen, & Quartz, 2008), particularly when perception of unfairness involves social comparisons with others (Fliessbach et al., 2007). In still another example, reward circuits of the striatum are activated when people are given an opportunity to punish cheaters. People appear to derive satisfaction from punishing norm violators rather than experiencing empathy for their pain (de Quervain et al., 2004)

Many empathy switches involve complex social reasoning and forethought. They involve neural circuits widely distributed throughout much of the brain. Ochsner et al. (2002) have shown how successful reappraisal of a social situation activates prefrontal cortex systems that focus attention, while deactivating the amygdala and associated circuits that normally alert to emotionally meaningful events. This sequence neutralizes negative affect generated by the social situation, which helps empathic processes to operate. Farrow et al. (2001) found that empathic judgments relative to social reasoning produced a complex pattern of brain activation that included the mirror neuron system, prefrontal executive functions systems, medial prefrontal systems for emotional perspective taking, and a posterior region of the cortex that coordinates orientation in space, visual gaze, and attentional systems. (See Figure 2.4.)

In summary, empathy switches produce top-down regulation of information processing that can reduce responsiveness of the pain matrix to others' suffering by compartmentalizing or suppressing inputs from the mirror neuron systems or by amplifying other competing streams of information. Some of these processes are explicit and conscious, whereas many others operate implicitly, automatically, and outside conscious awareness. Allocation of attention by the dorsal anterior cingulate and lateral prefrontal cortices and emotional perspective taking by the medial prefrontal cortex appear to play

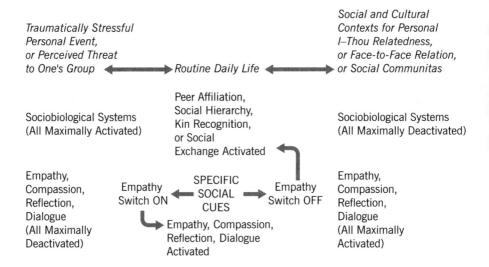

FIGURE 2.4. The sociobiological and neurobiological scope of religious life. Perceived events in routine daily life cue empathy switches that bring either sociobiological religion or processes of personal spirituality into dominance. Traumatically stressful life events or perceived threats to group identity can maximally activate sociobiological systems within religious life, while deactivating personal spirituality. Social and cultural contexts that promote I–Thou relatedness (Buber, 1958), a face-to-face relation (Levinas, 1961, 1981/1997), or social communitas (Turner, 1969, 1974, 1982) can maximally activate processes of personal spirituality while deactivating sociobiological systems in religious life.

key roles. Personal psychology, in terms of attachment relationships and self-identity, and social psychology, in terms of social identities and social dominance, set the categories for moral reasoning and bias the values that guide decision making. The involved neural pathways are evolutionarily engineered with their steps hardwired. However, empathy switches that send behaviors down one path or another are governed by beliefs, appraisals, and other psychological processes.

Withdrawal of Empathy
Can Open a Guilt-Free Zone for Aggression

Natural morality relies on a sustained capacity to feel the pain of others. When not empathically attuned, actions can be given freely to whatever seems most gratifying. The playing field is cleared of guilt or remorse. In a novel study of "altruistic punishment," de Quervain et al. (2004) utilized functional brain imaging to show how some people derive so much satisfaction from punishing others that they are willing to harm themselves in the process. In this PET scan study, subjects could punish defectors in a game either by a symbolic slap on the hand or by taking away money the defector would have received from participating. Some subjects were willing to deprive themselves of their own rewards, so much was their zeal to punish norm violators. These subjects showed heightened activation in the dorsal region of the striatum that promotes utility and efficiency (de Quervain et al., 2004), not empathic sensing of pain for those who were doled out punishment (Hsu et al., 2008; King-Casas et al., 2005).

Guilt is a social emotion that mobilizes a person to make restitution by "putting things right" with the person who was wronged. Functional withdrawal of empathy short-circuits guilt. If the other's pain is not experienced in the first place, then there is no felt need for restitution. It is thus typical for an aggressor to create a narrative that supports a functional withdrawal of empathy for the other. The justification can be moral, as when framing the other as a cheater or betrayer, or sociobiologically driven, as when discriminating against those low in status within one's group or those in outgroups who are deemed unworthy of empathy.

How Neurobiology Helps Make Sense of Harmful Religious Behaviors

The interaction between the social environment and the biological structure of the brain is in constant flux. As displayed in Figure 2.4, traumatic experiences and perceived threats to one's group can massively activate all sociobiological systems, while fully suppressing processes of personal spirituality, resulting in a "Praise God and pass the ammunition!" state of mind. Perceptions of others are in terms of social categories to which they belong and awareness of other as person is lost. At the other end of the spectrum, a committed opening of one's being within emotions of reverence, wonder, and concern maximally activates brain systems that support processes of spirituality, including reflection, dialogue, empathy, and compassion. The sociobiological systems then become quiescent, and cognitive processes are fully focused on the personhood of the other with loss of awareness of his or her social category, whether social status, ethnicity, gender, or religious group.

Most of the time, the sociobiology of religion operates in a midrange where emotional arousal is at manageable levels. The sociobiological systems then perform their maintenance functions of building and repairing group structures, whether families, organizations, communities, or societies. Social cues activate different sociobiological systems to respond differently to different people in different situations, according to the dictates of family, group, or societal roles and hierarchy.

Religion is at risk for harming people when it revolves around only its sociobiology and neurobiology, absent processes of personal spirituality. Empathic listening, empathy, moral reflection, compassion, and dialogue serve central roles in all spiritualities. Empathy is attenuated when brain circuits supporting these processes are deactivated. Empathy depends on robust explicit memory from the hippocampus and efficient executive functions from prefrontal cortex, both of which can become disorganized when there is sensory overload, emotional flooding, or a selective cutoff by an empathy switch. To be effective, interventions to counter harmful uses of religion must attend to the sociobiological and neurobiological contours of religious life. A neurobiological perspective can bolster the effectiveness of clinical interventions in any of four ways that occur commonly in interactions with patients.

First, a neurobiological perspective directs a clinician to prioritize the monitoring of nonverbal, bodily signs of emotions in order to guide what one does with language (Griffith & Griffith, 1994, pp. 65–93). Possibilities for dialogue are set by the physiological state of the brain, whose bias can favor either dialogue or debate, collaboration or confrontation. Patients who already feel under siege for their religious beliefs or practices enter clinical encounters physiologically primed for battle. Averted gaze, closed posture, tensed muscles, tight voice, and shallow breathing, for example, are signs that biological prerequisites for dialogue are missing. Nonverbal, bodily signs of hypervigilance can be more reliable indicators than a patient's words.

Rather than attempt to force dialogue that cannot easily happen, a clinician can focus instead on lowering perceptions of oneself as a threat and on interactions that do not press the patient into a vulnerable position. In fact, it is often more important to be perceived as nonthreatening than it is to offer a warm, kind, supportive relationship. Negative goodness, carefully avoiding threatening behaviors, can be of greater value than positive goodness when distrust is palpable.

Second, neurobiology points to an overriding importance that the global level of emotional arousal can hold. The limbic system of a patient's brain can resonate with the overall tone and intensity of emotions in a clinical interaction, more so than with details of verbal interchanges with a clinician. It is important to recognize when a patient has become emotionally flooded. A neurobiological perspective devotes maximal effort to learning about a patient's trip wires for alarm responses and strategizing how to avoid them.

Amygdala hyperarousal and defensive behaviors may run their own autono- mous course once initiated, often beyond the clinician's influence or even the patient's willpower. An unrepairable rupture in relationship is a risk. The time course for recovery from an alarm response can extend over hours or days, bare of openings through which reassuring words, soothing movements, or even apologies make much difference. Once out of the corral, one may simply have to wait for the horse to return.

Third, a neurobiological perspective suggests not attempting dialogue until it has been determined whether biological prerequisites for dialogue are present. Key questions for appraising possibilities for dialogue are: Does the patient feel safe? Does the patient feel secure? Does the patient feel respected? Speaking, listening, and reflecting, as well as dialogical processes of personal spirituality—whole-person relatedness, empathy, compassion, dialogue, moral reflection—all rely upon a neurophysiological infrastructure that goes offline during states of alarm from threat or uncertainty. Breathing and muscle relax- ation techniques, grounding techniques, guided imagery, and carefully paced interview questions are methods that trauma psychotherapists have developed to help patients with posttraumatic stress disorder to dearouse before attempt- ing to engage in dialogue about traumatic events (Rothschild, 2000, 2003; Griffith & Griffith, 1994). Clinicians can also encourage patients to utilize such spiritual resources as prayers, meditation, or recitation of sacred scrip- tures as ongoing practices that can help sustain a high-security/low-arousal state, which, in turn, enables better use of empathy, dialogue, and reflection in clinical encounters.

Finally, medications sometimes can be used to modify the physiological state of the brain to one more favorable to dialogue, reflection, empathy, and other processes that are central to personal spirituality. For the most part, pharmacological interventions are reserved for treatment of psychiatric disor- ders where there are fundamental impairments functioning in specific brain circuits, as is discussed in the final section of this text.

3

✦

Setting the Stage
Opening Dialogue about Religious Life

PATIENTS SELDOM SEEK HELP FROM MENTAL HEALTH CLINICIANS because they are putting their religion to use in harmful ways. Involvement of mental health clinicians usually arises when someone else becomes alarmed, for example, a pastor worried about a church member, an internist or pediatrician concerned about a patient's safety, an inpatient psychiatric unit alerted to suicide risk, an employer or school system frightened about an employee's or student's behavior, or a court intervening to protect a vulnerable family member. Involving a patient's religious life within a clinical treatment program might make sense throughout a course of medical or psychiatric treatment should it strengthen resilience or promote healing (Griffith & Griffith, 2002; Pargament, 2007). Addressing harmful uses of religion, however, is about devising interventions to protect against its potentially adverse effects in specific circumstances of concern. Often interventions must be conducted within a single or a handful of clinical encounters.

Addressing harmful uses of religion is an art that emphasizes the importance of improvised, stand-alone clinical conversations in which dialogue must be initiated under hostile conditions. Formal, contracted psychotherapy is too often an unrealistic expectation. A patient often does not view behaviors alarming others as problematic and has no wish to change. A clinician may need to work from an outgroup position as a scrutinized, distrusted, or even disliked "stranger." On religiously ideological grounds, a patient may view all secular mental health clinicians with disdain. Agreement to meet with the clinician may have come about only after some degree of coercion by whoever instigated the referral. The clinician likewise may struggle to respect the patient's religious identity. There often is no shared agreement between clinician and patient as to what would be a good outcome.

Under these circumstances, building dialogue that leads to successful therapeutic interventions requires conceptual frameworks and interview methods that may not be standard parts of many clinicians' repertoires in outpatient psychotherapy. Conceptually, a clinician needs a map that helps grasp the perspectives of persons doing harm via their religious or ideological commitments. This perspective taking may be possible at only a cognitive level at the start, but eventually must locate the patient's emotional perspective as well so that authentic empathy and compassion for the patient become KEY possible. Skilled perspective taking guides how a conversation is structured so that respectful listening and honoring the patient's dignity are paramount.

Put differently, a clinician must make psychological sense of a patient's perceptions, thoughts, feelings, and behaviors from within the patient's religious or ideological worldview, within its discourse, and using its own categories of meaning. Rapid assessment of involved sociobiological or neurobiological factors helps make the patient's perspectives more intelligible. Critical, moment-to-moment decision making is required to avoid triggering a patient's empathy switches, which can suddenly pull back any wish for relatedness with the clinician. With such an understanding, a clinician can take primary responsibility for positioning his/her self where dialogue may be most possible, standing close enough to the patient's world to be able to understand it but not so close as to pose a threat. From this position, a clinician can listen for the patient's unique language and practices of religious life that might provide a foundation on which further dialogue can be built.

The Impact of an Unfortunate Freudian Legacy

Conversations with patients about their religious lives can be challenging to initiate even when there are no concerns about harmful uses of religion. Through most of the 20th century, mutual distrust and stigmatizing judgments kept distance between religion and the professional disciplines of psychiatry and psychology. Sigmund Freud's attitude toward religion long held sway in keeping religion at an intellectual distance from the mental health disciplines. Psychoanalysis helped free sexuality from the moral judgments of an earlier age. However, it treated religion as a "black tide of mud" and a source of irrationality from which scientific practitioners aspired to lift mankind (Jung, 1963, pp. 150–151). At the peak of psychoanalytic influence, clinicians too interested in religion were viewed by colleagues as either unenlightened or troubled. This attitude limited serious discussion for a therapeutic role of religion. Moreover, the public, educated by movie portrayals and pop psychology, grew savvy about how mental health professionals viewed religion.

Although the American general population remained highly religious in their personal lives, most people understood that this was not a proper topic to raise with a psychiatrist, psychologist, or other mental health professional. Some physicians kept open an interest in the role of religion in coping with medical illnesses, but they were looked upon as unsophisticates by their mental health colleagues. So there grew through much of the 20th century a cultural consensus, involving both clinicians and their patients, that talk about religion was not appropriate for clinical conversations.

Religious people have expected to be belittled by mental health professionals and often avoided psychiatric treatment unless it was forced upon them by the severity of a family member's illness. Although this stigma has lessened recently, professional offices of psychiatrists and psychologists still are not natural settings for most patients to discuss intimate experiences of their religious lives.

Religion as a Stigmatized Discourse

Hesitation from fear of stigma can make clinical conversations about religion feel awkward to both clinician and patient. In ancient Greece, cuts or burns were placed on the bodies of disreputable people—slaves, criminals, traitors— so they could be easily recognized and avoided in public places. These physical stigmata identified a person as blemished (Goffman, 1963). Stigma still exists as a social construction that has two elements: (1) a "mark" as some publicly recognizable difference from other people; and (2) a consequent devaluation of the marked person (Dovidio, Major, & Crocker, 2000). The more publicly visible the mark, the better it can serve the role of stigma.

There is much about religious behavior that can serve admirably as a stigmatizing mark: a hijab, a crucifix, "Have a blessed day!" as a spontaneously spoken religious expression. Usually religious people are keenly aware whether public religious expression places them at risk for discrimination or humiliation. When in doubt, most who are religious discreetly cover obvious signs of their religious identities. Proselytizing religious groups who want maximal public visibility take advantage of this social process by encouraging adherents to announce their religious beliefs as loudly as possible. Religious faith that prizes private practices, for example, someone who conducts Buddhist meditative practices in the solitude of his or her home, is at little risk for stigma compared with a member of the Unification Church, who is robed and chanting outside the stairs to the subway.

Religious Countertransference as a Clinical Problem

Clinicians historically have contributed to stigma through assumptions that overtly religious behaviors indicated psychopathology and through emotional responses described as "religious countertransference." Religious countertransference refers to emotional responses toward a patient's religious language, beliefs, practices, rituals, or community that diminish the effectiveness of treatment (Griffith, 2006). Religious countertransference arises when a clinician begins reacting to a patient's religious expressions as though nothing more need be known about the patient as a person. Religious countertransference not only obstructs therapeutic relationships and obscures treatment options; it also demeans the humanity of the clinician. A clinician who in other settings might show compassion and awareness of a patient's uniqueness instead becomes emotionally distant and disinterested in an overtly religious patient.

Early psychoanalysts viewed countertransference narrowly as an unfortunate intrusion of a psychotherapist's own unresolved unconscious conflicts into the work of a psychotherapy (Slakter, 1987). In recent decades, countertransference in psychotherapy has been regarded more broadly to include normal human responses to patients' behaviors and attitudes (Winnicott, 1949). In this sense, countertransference describes the whole set of nontherapeutic emotional responses by clinicians toward their patients (Gabbard, 2000). These can include emotions stirred by patients who openly display, express, or enact their religious faiths during clinical encounters.

Religious countertransference has had multiple sources. Religious people have been regarded as opposed to science in their ignorance or, more pathologically, as making neurotic suffering seem honorable. Ethical concerns about imposing a clinician's values upon patients have served as justifications for avoiding any discussion of religious issues. Many clinicians have simply felt incompetent and preferred that patients would have such discussions with clergy or chaplains. This hovering cloud of stigma has made it difficult to hear the complexities of people's spiritual lives. It has pointed to the need for learning how to listen for a stigmatized discourse, one left unexpressed because of fears of humiliation.

Religion as Social Identity

Processes of stigma revolve around social identity. Religious commitment can be a core element of a person's social identity. Social identity is constituted by features of a person that permit others to anticipate what may be the person's social status, social category, and attributes (Goffman, 1963). A person can feel vulnerable when one's social identity is put center stage as a topic of conversation. As Erving Goffman (1967, p. 10) succinctly put it; "While his social face can be his most personal possession and the center of his security and pleasure, it is only on loan to him from society; it will be withdrawn unless he conducts himself in a way that is worthy of it." When a person's identity is met with respect, a door to intimacy is opened; when it is devalued, the person shrinks back in shame and humiliation.

For example, Mr. Jarvis, a patient who lived alone, suffered from failing vision and had a leg amputated as a result of complications of diabetes. Now he was facing congestive heart failure and further worsening of his disability. "Is religious faith important in your life?" I asked directly, wondering whether there might exist a community of faith that could respond to his loneliness and such practical needs as transportation to the grocery store or physical therapy. I learned that Mr. Jarvis had, in fact, been a long-standing member of a local Baptist church but had lost touch as friends and associates died or moved away. When contacted about his plight, the church fortunately responded by reengaging him in their outreach ministry for the elderly.

My greatest concern was a practical one: Mr. Jarvis urgently needed a community of support. Was there a chance, however, that my direct question about his religious faith might have felt offensive to Mr. Jarvis? There is, of course, always that chance. He might have wondered if I looked down upon Baptists. Had it been the case that he, in fact, followed no religion, he might have assumed I would judge him for being nonreligious. As a white psychiatrist asking an African American patient about his church, the question could have heightened awareness of racial differences between us. Asking a patient about his or her religious life is akin to asking about one's ethnicity, family background, or sexual identity. Imagine asking a new acquaintance at a dinner party, "Where did your people come from?" Perhaps some guests might be glad to be asked, but others would be circumspect until the reason for asking was clarified, and still others would be offended from the start by the question's intrusion into private space.

Clinicians' good intentions thus have their limitations. Whether a question about religious identity is experienced as empathic and affirming, or judging and scorning, depends largely upon factors outside the clinician's control: the social context of the interaction, how the patient perceives the clinician's intent, and the patient's cultural presuppositions of which the clinician may be unaware. The patient's experience of the question is the final arbiter of its ✓ meaning regardless how these factors fall. Unfortunately, ambiguity about the meaning of a question is often by default interpreted as ridicule when religion is the topic. This risk should be anticipated when mutual acknowledgments of respect have not yet been established in a treatment relationship.

Religion and Inchoate Experience

Unrelated to stigma, there is yet another reason why discussions about religion or spirituality can be difficult. Religious experience often exists inchoate. That is, religious experience is often remarkably difficult to put into words that are meaningful to another person. A clinician simply needs to respect how hard this can be.

Martin Buber observed that a relationship with a spiritual being "does not use speech, yet begets it. We perceive no Thou, but none the less we feel we are addressed and we answer—forming, thinking, acting" (Buber, 1958, p. 6). Spiritual experiences can be felt deeply as images or bodily sensations, powerful in moving a person to action, yet inexpressible in language. Explaining an intense religious experience to a person who has not had such an experience is perhaps akin to explaining what it is like to fall in love to a listener who has never been in love. It is hard to feel that even making the explanation is worth the effort. The religious patient does not bring it up, and the clinician often does not ask.

The Single Chance to Make a First Impression: Etiquette, Respect, and Sensitive Listening

How does one initiate dialogue with a patient who may be wary, defensive, and suspicious of a mental health professional's intentions? When doubts about the other already exist, chances for further relationship frequently turn on a first impression.

Commitment to attentive and respectful listening is the major priority. Attendees in workshops I have conducted over the years on psychotherapy and spirituality have often asked: "What are good questions to ask?" Preparing in advance some questions to ask can help quell a clinician's uncertainty. Yet learning to listen for referents to spirituality in the spontaneous flow of a clinical dialogue has been the most critical skill for initiating dialogue about spirituality. Listening, not asking, usually is the greater priority.

This listening must be conducted in a manner that is welcoming. It is the same active listening that would be needed to start an honest, frank conversation with a person belonging to any stigmatized group, such as those marked by race, sexual identity, or social class. A person at risk learns to become situation conscious, watching for subtle signs that indicate scrutiny or scorn, conscientiously editing what is shown to the other. As Erving Goffman (1963, p. 14) noted, a stigmatized person interacting with those outside one's own group "is likely to feel that he is 'on,' having to be self-conscious and calculating about the impression he is making, to a degree and in areas of conduct which he assumes others are not." Awareness of risks for stigmatization, including religious ones, tends to evoke similar social behaviors among people in marginalized groups:

+ Close editing of what is said in order "to be appropriate."
+ Vigilance for subtle signs of acceptance or rejection.
+ Keen sensitivity to power differences in the relationship.
+ When unsure, interpreting silence or ambiguous communications by default as disdain, contempt, scorn, or belittlement.

Ryszard Kapuscinski (2006, p. 35) has summarized this other-focused listening posture by referencing it to Emmanuel Levinas's philosophy of alterity: "If I fail to make the effort to notice or to show a desire to meet—we shall pass each other by indifferently, coldly and without feeling, blandly and heartlessly. Meanwhile, says Levinas, the Other has a face, and it is a sacred book in which good is recorded. Here our interest is in Levinas's thesis about the fundamental meaning of difference—that we accept the Other, although he is different, it is a good thing."

It is axiomatic that a person from the mainstream culture may find it difficult to notice the differences that matter most to a person from a marginalized culture. When unnoticed, these differences become obstacles to the openness that effective clinical work requires. An interviewing style that transcends these processes must strive to know the preferred identity of the other person by expressing interest in differences, not just commonalities, between the clinician and the person. Such an interviewing style is characterized by:

✦ Demonstrating explicit respect for the other.

✦ Indicating a desire to know the particularities of the other's experience.

✦ Listening for what may be difficult for the other to express.

✦ Avoiding a standard interview protocol, instead asking questions uniquely tailored out of curiosity and an authentic wish to know the other.

Such interview practices foster disclosure, rather than closeting, of spiritual life.

Fortunately, people across cultures can recognize each other's basic emotional expressions, including delight and disgust (Ekman, 2003). Expressions of delight free of disgust are the heart of showing respect. The safety necessary for openness must be signaled, no less an imperative when knowledge of the other's culture or language may be missing.

Hearing Language That Expresses Religious and Spiritual Experience

An empathic, flowing dialogue is aided by questions that inquire about patients' metaphors, stories, or beliefs as they are mentioned in the conversation. The clinician simply responds to what the patient has put on the table. For example, Ms. Fern, a large Jamaican woman, had for years been suffering from the constant pain associated with degeneration of multiple cervical and lumbar spinal disks. Despite the physical pain, she came across as a delightfully flamboyant person who loved visitors and conversation. "What helps you get through the bad days?" I asked. "My people and my God," she responded. I asked how a relationship with her God helped her cope with pain. She crossed her arms over her chest in a dramatic gesture and said, "When I pray to God, I have this warm feeling inside!" I wondered how this relationship with God was special compared with her human relationships. "When I tell something to God, I don't have to hear it again," she responded enthusiastically. "If I tell it to my girlfriend, then she tells it to this one, and this one tells it to that one, then I eventually hear it told to me. If I tell it to God, I never hear it again!"

This was an easy conversation. Ms. Fern's religion was so much in the everyday flow of her life that not to ask about it might seem odd. Moreover, she was not conflicted by any threat of stigma. Culturally, that simply was not part of her world. Yet I have noted, during years of teaching students and psychiatry residents, how many would seem not to hear her phrase "and my God" and inquire about it. Rather, they would pass over it to the next clinical question about symptoms or her psychiatric history. For Ms. Fern, this phrase pointed to a secure attachment with her God that helped sustain her through suffering.

Dialogue about spirituality mostly consists of listening for and inquiring about referents to religion and spirituality as they appear naturally in conversations. Religious experience can be presented as idioms, metaphors, narratives (stories), beliefs, prayers (or other intrapersonal dialogues with nonmaterial beings), spiritual practices, rituals and ceremonies, religious or spiritual communities, and daily practices of ethical living (Griffith & Griffith, 2002). It is important to listen broadly for any of these, because some forms are emphasized in particular religious traditions more so than others. For example, many Protestant Christians in North America rely most upon religious beliefs, the study of the Bible as a sacred scripture, and private prayer with a personal God. However, religious beliefs can play a less central role within Hinduism or Buddhism, where spiritual practices—meditation, dietary practices, chanting—serve more central roles. The point is that well-practiced, disciplined listening for any of these symbolic forms prepares a clinician to attend to a person's unique spirituality and experiential world (Griffith & Griffith, 2002). A brief review of these expressive forms can clarify their roles in listening.

Listening for Religious Idioms

To start, an idiom is a shorthand expression that has salient meaning within a particular subculture. Use of an idiom identifies a person as a member of that subculture. Idioms proliferate within such groups as teenagers, football teams, and military units, who want to establish a strong sense of shared identity and separateness from those outside the group.

Religious groups often use their particular idioms to mark the group boundary. When noticed by a clinician, a question about the expression can serve as a portal into a deeper conversation about the person's religious identity. Such a question can catch the person off guard: Idioms are usually spoken in a manner that suggests nothing further needs to be stated. Mr. Miller, for example, a man in his 60s, was chronically ill and in pain from pancreatitis. When asked how his spirits were in dealing with the illness, he responded, "God has prepared a place." "Can you tell me about the place?" I asked. Mr. Miller seemed momentarily surprised and then began telling me in more detail how tired he was from living each day with a diseased body, that God did not want him to suffer, and God had prepared a "place with many mansions" where suffering was forgotten. He thus treated me as a guest to whom he was willing to reveal private images from his religious faith.

"Praise God!", "I prayed for God's mercy," and "Oh, God help me!" are examples of religious idioms that often are spoken in a matter-of-fact manner, yet can open into serious dialogue about religious faith if a serious inquiry is made.

Listening for Metaphors of God or Spirituality

Metaphors are the evocative images that people use when trying to grasp the ineffable essence of God, other nonmaterial beings, or spirituality itself. They are evocative because they draw from familiar, well-trodden human experiences in an effort to articulate how the spiritual realm might similarly operate.

Several years ago, a research study with colleagues at the University of Mississippi Medical Center interviewed people about experiences of transcendence in their lives (Polles et al., 1993; Griffith et al., 1995; Griffith & Griffith, 2002). Each of these research participants had indicated on a questionnaire that God was "like a heavenly father," but further conversation with each revealed more poignant metaphors. They found their God to be:

+ "Like a warm cocoon, enclosing me as the world falls in around me."
+ "Like an exasperated mother whom I have disappointed and been ungrateful to too often."
+ "Like a nourishing, flowing river that comes to me, the parched dry river bed, and gives me life."
+ "Like a strict old grandfather, angry with my continual wrongdoing, who has finally turned his back on me."
+ "Like a nursing mama who is happy to be close to me and always has plenty of milk. As I lay my head on her breast, I feel her breathing and hear her heartbeat and I am calmed."

Hearing the metaphors that a person uses for God or spirituality gives the listener some idea of what will be likely qualities of that person's religious experiences. They often point toward expectations for relationships, whether with God, others in a religious group, or those outside the group.

Listening for Narratives of Religious Experience

A narrative is a story or episode from one's lived experience. A narrative has characters and a plot. It describes a sequence of events, both objective and subjective, happening within the consciousness of the characters: their fears, aspirations, doubts, and decisions (White, 2007). Unlike metaphors that are timeless (e.g., "God [was, is, and always will be] my heavenly father"), a narrative has a beginning, a middle, and an end: For example, "I remember the moment when I most felt close to God. . . ."

Narratives make individual events of a person's life comprehensible by locating where they lie within the larger scope of a person's life (Polkinghorne, 1988). Narratives shape what can be noticed, what can be thought about, and what actions are reasonable to consider. One can think of the self as constituted by important first-person narratives. Mr. Chin, in the Introduction, told narratives of his suffering in China during the persecution of the Fulan Gong, imprisonment and expulsion from his country, and a religious faith and community that helped him to prevail. He told narratives about seriously ill Fulan Gong members who had been miraculously healed through their spiritual practices. Lying in a hospital bed with a fractured hip, these narratives influenced him to reject his orthopedic surgeon's treatment recommendations.

It was through his narratives that Mr. Chin clarified how his Fulan Gong faith provided not simply a social role and community of support but also his personal sense of purpose and his relationship with the sacred. Whether or not I agreed with Mr. Chin's decision about surgery, I could make sense of it after hearing his stories. Hearing a person's narratives is perhaps the broadest opening through which to gain clarity about a person's religious life.

Listening for Religious Beliefs

A belief is a propositional statement that asserts what is real or what is important. Beliefs are typically drawn from or are justified by narratives from one's experiences in living. Mr. Chin's beliefs about the Fulan Gong way were thus directly related to the narratives he told. Beliefs can be also drawn from other authoritative sources, such as scientific research, political ideologies, and Internet websites. Religious beliefs are commonly derived from sacred texts, such as the Upanishads, the Qur'an, or the Bible, or from the teachings of religious leaders.

Clinically, beliefs matter not for their truth but for their consequences. Religious beliefs are often mistaken as scientific hypotheses because both are posed as propositional statements. Unlike scientific hypotheses, religious beliefs do not rest upon evidence for their validity, and absence of evidence rarely leads to their being discarded. Rather, beliefs are regarded as valid when they help people sustain morale—existential postures of hope, purpose, and port such existential postures.

Beliefs are also valid when they help maintain cohesion within one's religious group. For Mr. Chin, beliefs about the Fulan Gong were the most important source of hope and purpose in his life. They also drew him close to other members of his religious community. The fact that medical science did not support his beliefs about the curative power of his spiritual practices had no bearing upon their validity as religious beliefs.

Neurobiologically, beliefs often represent models of reality stored in implicit, or nondeclarative, memory. Implicit memories appear as feelings, images, or bodily sensations, with no felt sense of remembrance (Siegel, 1999). As such, people commonly do not experience these implicit models as beliefs, but rather as gut feelings, intuitions, or prejudices about "how the world really is."

Unlike idioms, metaphors, or narratives, beliefs often imply relationships of power between people. That which is believed to be real or important puts limits upon rights and privileges of other people (Griffith & Griffith, 2002). This accounts for the old adage that politics and religion—both belief laden—should be avoided as topics for polite conversations. Beliefs commonly are used to regulate religious group boundaries, distinguishing who is in or out of the group and determining who has access to what information. Beliefs are also used to enforce social hierarchies within religious groups, including group members' relations with their leaders.

Discussion of religious beliefs easily turns into a minefield in which tenuous alliances for treatment explode. This is particularly so when a patient belongs to a fundamentalist religious faith regardless of type. Adherence to specific beliefs in fundamentalist faiths often is a primary source for personal identity, group cohesion, and group boundary regulation. A more pragmatic strategy is to inquire about personal stories that in important ways give form to the patient's religious faith rather than asking what he or she believes to be ultimate truths.

Listening for Prayers or Other Intrapersonal Religious Dialogues

Psychologist Mary Watkins (1986, p. 1) has commented: "In the Hebraic tradition human beings were distinguished from all other living creatures not by virtue of their capacity for reason but by virtue of their engagement with three kinds of dialogues: dialogues with neighbors, with themselves, and with God." As far into our human history as scholarship can reach, human beings not only perceived and reacted to gods but also conversed regularly with them, publicly and privately.

These person-to-God conversations bear many resemblances to person-to-person conversations. However, some differences are also distinctive (Griffith & Griffith, 1994, 2002). Conversations with God typically assume implicitly that:

+ *God knows all.* There are no secrets in a relationship with God.
+ *God can be always present and available.* Humans, despite best efforts, cannot promise this.
+ *God is an eternal witness to a person's life and the final arbiter of justice.*
+ *Conversation with God commonly requires little spoken language.* Prayers directed toward God often are quite loquacious. However, God's responses most often are felt viscerally and nonverbally, sparse in words. Compared with most human conversations, a prayerful dialogue with God can be notably nonverbal.

These unique aspects of person-to-God dialogues mean that they can serve emotional roles for attachment that human relationships sometimes cannot. For example, God's knowledge of a person's most private thoughts surpasses what any other person can know. The felt intimacy of a relationship with God, both in closeness and in constancy, can transcend the intimacy of any human relationship.

However, dialogues with God can go awry as can human ones, particularly if there is an insecure attachment with God. The character of prayers to God then becomes stagnant, empty, and devoid of creative inspiration, attempting more to placate or complain to God than to engage in authentic dialogue. It is sometimes helpful for a clinician to ask questions that elaborate the characterization of God and foster interest in God's complexity as a psychological being who has feelings, intentions, concerns, and even ambivalence (Griffith & Griffith, 2002).

Listening for Spiritual Practices

Spiritual practices—meditation, dietary practices, chanting, recitation of sacred scriptures—transform a person through prescribed and repetitive actions. As Wittgenstein noted, "We reach the end of doubt, rather in practice. Children do not learn that books exist, that armchairs exist—they learn to fetch books, sit in armchairs" (cited in Monk, 1991, p. 578). A spiritual practice repeats the same actions, occasion after stereotyped occasion, engaging body and mind simultaneously.

Socially, the performance of a specific spiritual practice signals to others the identity of a person's particular religious tradition. Adherence to specific spiritual practices can serve as an important component of a person's social identity. Spiritual practices play central roles in Buddhism, Hinduism, and postmodern spiritualities. In some of these traditions, religion may not center upon the vicissitudes of a relationship with a personal God. Rather, awareness, knowledge, and ethical living are priorities, and adherence to spiritual practices is a primary method for attaining them (Griffith & Griffith, 2002; Griffith & Dsouza, in press).

Listening for Rituals

Rituals share with spiritual practices their character as prescribed, patterned actions. Rituals provide humans with practical methods for experiencing directly the numinous. Anthropologist Victor Turner (1982, p. 79) concluded from his studies that this is a core element of rituals: "A ritual is prescribed formal behavior for occasions not given over to technological routine, having reference to beliefs in invisible beings or powers regarded as the first and final causes of all effects." A ritual provides an experience of the holy—wonder, awe, joy—by structuring a meeting place where a person can touch the supernatural. A religious ritual is thus associated with creative change and emotions of wonder, awe, and openness to new possibilities. This distinguishes it from compulsive "rituals" that represent psychopathology and a form of anxiety disorder. Rituals are typically associated with the major myths and sagas of a religion, enabling a direct encounter between bodily experience and these culturally shaped myths and sagas (Griffith & Griffith, 2002).

Listening for Religious Communal Life

Each of these forms of symbolic expression has a social dimension that is expressed in roles and responsibilities within a religious group and in specifications for how relationships are to be conducted with those outside the religious group. Metaphors, stories, and beliefs are articulated in conversations with other people. Spiritual practices and rituals help create boundaries for communities of the faithful. What is distinctive about religious communities is that they can include nonmaterial beings. A "spiritual community" is constituted by both human and nonmaterial beings—God, angels, spirits, ancestors, saints—who can be engaged in concerned dialogue about problems. As Jesus told his disciples, "For where two or three are gathered in my name, there am I in the midst of them" (the Holy Bible, revised standard version, Matthew 18:20). One listens for these complex forms of communal life in order to understand a patient's participation in them.

Listening for Ethical Commitments

There are many who disavow any religious identity yet live disciplined lives that advance justice and compassion for others. For such a person, the idea of God is a distraction from what matters most: the truth about how one should live. Awareness of an implicit moral order is more compelling than the idea of God. A patient's ethical commitments articulate his or her sense of social exchange and reciprocal altruism within an ordered universe.

Opening a Generative Dialogue

The specific forms that an individual relies upon to express spirituality usually provide multiple portals through which a generative dialogue can be initiated. Such a dialogue can encourage the curiosity, openness, and reflection needed for creativity and change. Two contrasting vignettes, one with a religious patient and the other with a nonreligious patient, illustrate how this listening can open dialogue:

Mr. Duquesnay had been admitted for a neurological evaluation because of seizures that could not be controlled with medications (Griffith & Griffith, 1994, pp. 94–111). However, the seizures had proved to be stress-related symptoms, and not epileptic. A psychiatric evaluation helped to identify some of the factors in the patient's life that were aggravating his symptoms. As a result of his mother-in-law's illness, his wife wanted to move back to their hometown. However, Mr. Duquesnay had been sexually assaulted there as a child and had vowed never to return. Now he wanted to respond to his wife's request but could not bear facing the memories. Using his metaphor, he had been "burdened" by these events to the point that he began having somatic symptoms. As his dilemma had been revealed and openly discussed with his family, his symptoms ceased. He described the change as his "burden being lifted." After discharge home, however, he and his family realized they would need to manage these circumstances differently to prevent the burdening from building up again.

"When you feel unburdened," I asked, "what do you know about yourself as a person that you did not know before?" "That I am someone who is dedicated to living," he responded.

I took note of his words. "You know yourself as one who is dedicated to living?" I restated. "Yes, sir. I believe so," Mr. Duquesnay said. "I always have been that way. . . . The things that have piled up on me have taught me . . . like it did here."

"You have been burdened by so many things that all the burdens have covered up your being able to show yourself as one who is dedicated to living?" I responded, clarifying and underscoring his metaphor.

"You harden yourself," his wife interjected. "You're scared to let go because if you let go, you feel like you will go all to pieces. . . . So you just harden yourself against it all." "I think so," Mr. Duquesnay agreed.

"I think some of the more important questions for me to ask this morning have to do with the coming time after you are out of the hospital, back at home, back in your regular life. How do you prevent the burdening from building again? How to prevent how the old patterns—the old ways of living—from seducing you back under their influence. That is something I thought I should talk about, not just with you, but with the whole family. I figured that would be a family project."

"The number one thing is for there to be a difference in our prayer life and living for God. That's the number one thing. . . . And greater unity between us, understanding one another," Mr. Duquesnay answered.

I had expected that he would tell how he learned that more openness was needed in their family communications. I was startled by the response he gave instead, but followed his redirection.

"Well, tell me how the prayer life would work," I asked. "If I ask you to give the details. . . . How would you do it differently?"

"Well, I would have a much greater prayer life as a family. . . . I've never really had a prayer life with my family. . . . It's always been just me," Mr. Duquesnay responded.

"Prayer has been a private thing for you? But now you would want them to be a part of it?" I asked. "I think so. My wife has always tried to get it that way," Mr. Duquesnay said. "So Mrs. Duquesnay has already had that idea before that this would be good?" I asked.

"Right," Mr. Duquesnay responded, which prompted his wife to begin shaking her head. "Why are you shaking your head?" I asked Mrs. Duquesnay.

"Yeah. I've tried before to get him to let us. You know what they say: A family that prays together stays together. It's something I've felt like would benefit us all," Mrs. Duquesnay answered. "Because it is hard to stay mad at somebody . . . or if things go wrong, and if you are praying together . . . I don't know. He's always been a very private person."

"So you have seen prayer as a protection against the building up of burdens?" I asked Mrs. Duquesnay. "I think it helps," she responded. "We've been in church for a long time. When our prayer life is up, our troubles are less. But when we quit praying, everything seems to start falling apart around here. Or maybe when you get enough peace from God, you learn how to deal with it differently. I don't know."

"Was it down during the time before you came into the hospital?" I asked her. Mrs. Duquesnay laughed, shaking her head, "It's been down for a while!" Her husband and children nodded in unison. "Everybody agrees?" I asked. "They agree," Mr. Duquesnay responded. "They're laughing about it. They agree."

"How would you actually do that? Are you talking about having a prayer time together as a family?"

Mrs. Duquesnay told a story from her family when she was growing up. "That's really the number one thing," she said. "We love our church." She then told a story about the support their church community had provided to each other in the past.

This interview was a family interview on the day of discharge from the hospital. I believed that changes in their family interactions had been instrumental in Mr. Duquesnay's dramatic improvement. I had been frankly hoping for a direct discussion of these changes. Instead, the conversation took a different, but natural, turn toward their religious life when I asked them what had made a difference: "How do you prevent the burdening from building again?"

The story of religious life in the Duquesnay family unfolded as an account of Mr. Duquesnay's conflict between his personal spirituality and care of self and his sociobiological religious commitments to family. These conflicts were articulated with increasing specificity as an open family dialogue was facilitated.

"Burdening," "harden yourself," "prayer life," "the family that prays together stays together," "our church"—these words were ones that would stand out to a trained ear. There were referents to the religious life of the Duquesnay family. Each would provide a portal through which a well-crafted question might open a rich dialogue about their religious life. Each would point to a distinct domain of religious life with unique possibilities for contributing to comfort and health. Each also would contain within it unique risks for exacerbating suffering and illness.

With these words, members of the Duquesnay family explained the religious significance of what had happened during this family crisis and hospitalization. Their metaphors and stories provided maps for noticing what mattered most to them, what they considered as possibilities for change, and what actions might be needed if change were possible. I wondered as I listened:

✦ When did "burdening" first begin in Mr. Duquesnay's life? What events set the stage for it to happen? Why had it been a process so difficult to stop? What did Mr. Duquesnay believe that God understood about his life that he felt people in his life did not? Did he believe that God wanted him to be unburdened? What steps would God expect him to take to accomplish this?

✦ What did Ms. Duquesnay sense happened within her husband when she felt he "hardened himself?" What did she imagine were her husband's concerns? What did she imagine as God's involvement in this process? What steps did she believe God expected her husband to take? What steps did God expect her to take in helping him?

✦ When speaking about "our church," who was in that community? Was it the entire membership or a smaller group? How did church as a community matter? For whom in the family did it matter most? What might be the role of the church in a plan to prevent burdening to build up again for Mr. Duquesnay?

I noted that "prayer life" and "the family that prays together stays together" had been operating quite differently for Mr. and Mrs. Duquesnay as blueprints for how they each constructed personal and social realities. For Mr. Duquesnay, prayer had been an intimate and private conversation between him and his God; for Mrs. Duquesnay, prayer was a shared activity for bonding family members and buffering conflicts. There was tension between the spouses over which kind of prayer took priority. *NB*

This discussion also pointed beyond the field of family interaction to Mr. Duquesnay as a moral decisionmaker. Mr. Duquesnay sensed the different pulls: to be a husband in roles and behaviors that God and his church expected or to care first for himself as a person. This tension was enacted in his avoiding or accepting the traumatic memories that he feared he could not manage. No perfect choice lay before him. What, for Mr. Duquesnay, would constitute a good choice, one made in awareness of differing, potentially contradictory moral imperatives but keeping fidelity with the person he most hoped to be? How might a clinician provide consultation to Mr. Duquesnay to help him act more competently and effectively as a moral agent in his religious life?

The Secular Position of the Clinician

The interview with the Duquesnay family displays the secular role of a clinician when discussing religion in clinical encounters. Some assume there is an advantage to sharing with a patient a jointly held religious tradition. A shared tradition can provide a clinician with an insider's knowledge about a person's particular religious metaphors and beliefs. Sometimes this is an advantage, yet sometimes it is not. A listener with no familiarity often is better positioned for asking questions of authentic curiosity from a "not knowing" stance (Anderson, 1997). Such questions are often better invitations for the person to teach the listener details that are commonly passed over when a common understanding is assumed. When one, however, knows the religious tradition firsthand, this understanding of a metaphor within the faith's fabric of meanings can stimulate more nuanced questions. My insider's knowledge about the Duquesnay family's culture was partial. Although not sharing their Pentecostal Christian faith, I did know from my southern Mississippi childhood some of the rich religious histories of "burdening" and "hardening yourself" that I expected to be intimately familiar to the Duquesnay family. First, the Lamb of God taking on the burden of a person's sin is an image that runs through the New Testament scriptures. Second, the story of the Exodus describes the Hebrew people's struggle when "the heart of Pharaoh was hardened" (Exodus 9:35). I could be confident that these metaphors were evocative within the Duquesnay family's awareness. I could step into their use of their language with an ease that perhaps would not have been available to someone more culturally distant. However, such a person might have asked thoughtful questions about the meanings of these metaphors that plausibly could have opened a more therapeutic dialogue than would mine.

Listening for Spirituality
Not Centered in a Formal Religion

The story of Ms. Carlson stands in contrast to that of Mr. Duquesnay. It shows how listening proceeds when a person's spirituality is centered upon a sensed relational and moral order, but not a relationship with a personified God. Ms.

Carlson began a psychotherapy session by telling how she had been "running with every fiber of my being" since the last session after I asked her directly about her history of trauma. She had told me about a man who exposed himself to her on an elevator when she was 11 years old. Bystanders found her crying and called the police. When her father arrived home, however, he was furious that the police had been called. One of the policemen confronted her father because he appeared not to have been attending to his daughter. She turned immediately and defended her father to the policeman, even though she recalled inwardly feeling that "I wanted to scream and scream and scream!"

As Ms. Carlson recollected this memory, I asked her what was happening within her body. "Nothing," she said.

I changed the question. "You may be feeling nothing. But if you were to imagine your body right now getting ready to act in some way, or to express something, what would that be?"

"To hide and to scream!" she responded. "It's just chaos, all chaos. . . ."

"Do you remember what would bring comfort when you found yourself in that chaos as a little girl?" I asked.

"I would eat candy," she said. "I was an overeater. I was in Overeaters Anonymous for a decade, and it was helpful. But as I began settling down, food stopped being important to me." She recalled how candy would bring such calmness that she would keep it at her bedside, even though she no longer would actually eat it.

"At first Overeaters Anonymous was a safe place to be," she said. "A lack of judgment. You can say anything you want to say about yourself with understanding. You were free to feel your emotion." Her participation in OA ended during a time of heartbreak with the termination of a love affair. She talked about it within her OA group but felt she only received "slogans and a cant." She then began viewing OA as "robotic, unreal." "It was over. It was unreal. I felt alone again."

I commented upon her questioning, challenging, and critiquing, skeptical of promises people and groups made, yet clearly also yearning for relationships and community. I asked what she had found in her life that had proved solid.

She told how she had become passionately involved in the early women's movement. She founded one of the first legal abortion clinics in America. Her work with abortion led to a project in which she produced a manual on family planning, which was eventually published in four languages. She founded health coalitions in south Asia and Africa. She recalls her deepest meaning in the health and education projects she conducted in Bangladesh. Later she founded an international women's advocacy organization, which brought her to Washington, DC. She led it for several years, until she lost her leadership position during political infighting within the organization. "When it ended, I was 2 years in mourning," she recalled. She then became a journalist and editor. I asked whether this might have been the closest she had come to finding a community she could trust.

"Yes," she replied.

I asked whether it was the case then that she had found good people she could trust. "Yes. But I'm cut off from them right now. The only fun I've had at this job has been with writing some of the 'edge pieces.'"

I reviewed with her the outline of her life story as she had recounted it: her experiences with her angry father, her disappointments in relationships, assaults she had suffered. I could easily have imagined that she would become cynical or despairing. Yet she instead carried forward a resilient determination to live fully and to make the world a better place for others. What accounted for this?

She told how she was present at the bedside of her father when he died. "I saw him filled with a radiance . . . like yellow. . . . I experienced my father as freed, without his anger and torment." She paused, then added, "But I am not a religious person." Yet this moment at her father's deathbed had proven to be a pivotal event in her life that would help her stay free from the destructive influences of his anger and torment.

Ms. Carlson had been referred to me in her last years of her life when she suffered multiple medical illnesses. It was not unusual for her to arrive at a session in the company of a friend who came out of concern that she was not taking proper care of herself. It stood out repeatedly how much she was beloved. After her death, an outpouring of friends and those she had mentored told fond story after story about their time with her. She was remembered with devotion.

As we listen to Ms. Carlson's story, where do we hear her spirituality? Oddly, the first clue came from her thoughts as a child: "It's just chaos, all chaos." The metaphor of "chaos" marked her childhood hell. We then look later in the narrative to find a metaphor standing in apposition: "I experienced my father as freed, without his anger and torment." Her metaphor of apposition is implicit and not verbalized: It is one of liberation. People are not destined for chaos. Reality does not have to be chaotic. People and reality can be liberated. Her guiding image was the face of her dying father, filled with yellow radiance, liberated.

Next, we can ask whether she retreated before the chaos or stood against it. And if she stood against it, how? Her confrontation with chaos was decisive. Her method was to immerse herself in a community of women responding to those who were the weakest, suffered the most, and were most vulnerable. This community of gender cut across social, political, and national groups. When, as with OA, the community became formulaic, she moved on to new relationships that were vibrant and passionate.

Ms. Carlson was not religious. Yet she gave us this account of her spirituality: her metaphors of chaos and liberation, a narrative of her father's transformation, and her commitment to spirituality-in-community. If she were with us now, we might imagine what additional questions, when posed through these portals, might open yet more expansively a discussion of her spirituality:

+ In the midst of the childhood chaos, what, or who, kept alive the idea that liberation from chaos was possible?
+ If she could imagine her father in his last moments, freed of anger and torment, gazing upon her, what might he have hoped for her life? If he were able from an afterlife to witness her work with the women in Asia and Africa, what might have been his response?
+ What had she learned about the practical know-how for finding community in a world of chaos? When had she first appreciated that this could be a possibility? Who helped her discover this?

The progression of Ms. Carlson's life also can be told in terms of the steps she took to become a competent and effective moral agent, as she followed her commitment to liberate those beset by chaos, oppression, and hatred, while resisting pulls from family, organizations, and culture to live a more conventional life.

Managing Religious Countertransference: From Suppression to Perspective Taking to Exuberance

The listening illustrated in the stories of Mr. Duquesnay and Ms. Carlson only becomes possible when a clinician can open his or her emotional awareness fully to the presence of the patient as a person. This is difficult unless one can manage effectively any judgmental, disdainful, or hostile feelings that spontaneously may be evoked by a patient's particular brand of religiousness. For some clinicians, recollections of negative personal encounters with religion make treatment of explicitly religious patients frustrating and tiring. This is particularly so when childhood religious experiences or teachings were disturbing, painful, or simply boring. As when other kinds of personal experiences resonate disconcertingly, negative countertransference toward particular religious patients or their stories calls for self-reflection, self-awareness, and sometimes peer consultation or personal psychotherapy.

Sometimes, however, a clinician who is nonreligious simply feels incompetent when a patient brings spiritual or religious concerns into treatment. Feelings of incompetence stem from a misunderstanding for how professional skills of most mental health clinicians can aid a person struggling with a religious problem (Griffith & Griffith, 2002). Mental health clinicians bear competencies different from those of a pastor, priest, rabbi, or other religious professional. For example, diagnostic skills for identifying major psychiatric disorders can be helpful for a patient who confuses a major depressive disorder with normal grief or the intrusive thoughts of obsessive–compulsive disorder with normal guilt. Skills in working with relational conflicts can be applied as usefully to a person's conflicted relationship with his or her God as with human relationships.

Most problematic, however, is internalized professional stigma toward religion that is enacted through a clinician's assumptions, attitudes, and emotional availability (Griffith, 2006). An understanding of religious life from the perspectives of neurobiology, cognitive psychology, and social psychology can go a long distance toward helping a clinician to experience patients' religious expressions with curiosity and interest. Clinical illustrations in Chapters 5 through 8 illustrate how neurobiological and sociobiological perspectives can help attenuate negative religious countertransference.

When stigma is the issue, the therapeutic task is to rehumanize the patient within the clinician's consciousness. This means finding ways to experience the patient as a complex human being rather than as a thin character constituted only by his or her religious expression. The antidote for stigma is authentic expression of respect for the person. The challenge for a clinician is to relate to a patient in a way that respects his or her dignity. Clinical treatment that is open to dialogue about religious experience is often distinguished not so much by its religious content as by its similarities to clinical work with patients who, for other reasons, have been misunderstood or excluded by a dominant culture, whether by race, ethnicity, sexual identity, or economic status (Griffith, 2006).

When interviewing religious patients, it helps to adopt default therapeutic assumptions that sustain curiosity and respect for the other. One can embrace as operational truths such maxims as "the person is not the belief" or "off-putting public religion can hide personal spirituality." Pragmatically, these assumptions promote an emotional posture more likely to realize potentials for dialogue.

Deconstructive questions can open conversations that dissipate countertransferential feelings. Deconstructive questions make explicit the interpretive assumptions from which a particular religious belief emerged. This inquiry identifies these interpretive assumptions and delineates their cultural origins (White, 1995, 2007; Griffith & Griffith, 2002, pp. 151–155). A religious belief can then be viewed in a particular historical context and situated within a particular cultural discourse. These questions often shift the focus from a debate about truth or falsehood of a belief to understanding the person who holds it. Useful deconstructive interviewing strategies include:

+ Learning about the history of the person's religious beliefs and practices: "What were some events in your life that made this belief become important for you? What else was happening in your life while these events were occurring? How do these experiences contribute to how you think about and prioritize concerns now?"
+ Learning how religious beliefs or practices constitute the person's social identity: "With whom do you share this belief? From whom would you be separated if this belief were to change?"

Managing religious countertransference means meeting a patient as a person, not as a category. If this is successfully accomplished, possibilities for reflective dialogue can begin to open. There then is a chance for frank discussions about a patient's religious beliefs and practices as they relate to a clinical problem.

With time and practice, competencies for managing negative responses to patients' religiousness can mature. At the outset, stoic silencing of aversion to religious talk, styles of dress, or manners of relating may be the most that can be mustered for meeting minimal standards of courtesy and professionalism. However, self-silencing of aversion is arduous and exhausting. Accurately grasping cognitive and emotional perspectives of the patient's experience goes further toward building curiosity and interest so that aversion does not arise. When the otherness of a strangely different religious patient can be personally sensed, then interest and intrigue build, and even emotions of wonder and exuberance may be experienced. It is intrinsically gratifying to meet that within another person which cannot be understood but only responded to (Levinas, 1981/1997; Kapuscinski, 2006). Clinical encounters then produce rather than consume emotional energy.

The Outgroup Clinician:
Listening as an Outsider with a Visitor's Pass

Quieting the emotional static of religious countertransference permits listening to proceed. A clinician still must stay mindful of reasons that might render a patient reticent to speak about religion, particularly fears that he or she could be treated in a ridiculing or condescending manner. It helps when a clinician can be both imaginative and courageous: imaginative in perceiving how a patient who lives in a remote religious or ideological fiefdom perceives and thinks about the world, courageous in entering as fully as possible into his or her emotional experiences (Weingarten, 1995).

If one listens well and with respect, a clinician receives a "visitor's pass" to enter the patient's religious life, to meet its personages, and to view its landscape. A clinician can ask permissible questions, which can include questions at times that are remarkably intimate. However, a visitor's pass does not make one a citizen of the patient's realm. There are rights and privileges predictably not permitted. One may not, for example, be permitted to criticize explicitly the ruler or the laws of the realm. Mindfulness of the many forms through which religion and spirituality are expressed can aid this listening. This listening and mindfulness together set a stage where dialogue can become possible.

4

✦

Locating Personal Spirituality through Existential Inquiry

PERSONAL SPIRITUALITY IS RELIGION FOR THE PERSON. ITS BEACON is a person's desire and need for solace, comfort, and joy. Personal spirituality operates outside the dominion of sociobiology. It strengthens and cares first for individuals, not groups. Locating threads of personal spirituality within the complexly patterned fabric of religious life is an essential step when helping a patient to position religion on the side of health and healing.

Clinical assessment often begins by determining whether practical concerns about harm from a patient's religious life are, in fact, warranted and, if so, what factors contribute to the risks of harm. This assessment optimally is conducted within a collaborative dialogue that examines how different contributions to religious life come from personal spirituality, sociobiological religion, or, less commonly, psychiatric illness. Such a clinical dialogue needs to navigate past obstacles of religious stigma and counterstigma in order to find a relational position close enough for dialogue but not so close as to threaten. These steps are ones of watching and listening. Questions then can be asked about the patient's religious experience as it is typically expressed. Learning where personal spirituality is manifest within the broad scope of a patient's

81

life is of key importance. Existential questions are the primary clinical tools for this inquiry.

Existential Questions

Existential questions inquire how a person responds to the struggles and sorrows of everyday existence. Existential questions provide a safe and reliable path for learning about personal spirituality (Griffith & Gaby, 2005; Griffith & Dsouza, in press). They usually are experienced as normalizing, rather than pathologizing, because they ask about similar dark places through which all people, including the clinician, eventually walk.

In speaking with Ms. Johnson (see Introduction), I asked, "From where do you draw strength to get through a time like this?" My question was about her experience of living with a debilitating medical illness. She responded, "God and my friends," even though the question itself was not explicitly about religious faith. My question asked how she as a person responded to challenges she faced; it did not ask for the kinds of factual data that typically are used to categorize religious people: whether she regarded herself as religious, what were her religious beliefs, or whether be she belonged to a particular religious congregation. Such information would be a less useful guide to the heart of her spirituality.

Existential questions help articulate a person's spirituality by inquiring about personal encounters with adversity. Primo Levi recorded his observations about those who suffered with him in the Nazi death camp at Auschwitz: "Every human being possesses a reserve of strength whose extent is unknown to him, be it large, small, or nonexistent, and only through extreme adversity can we evaluate it" (1988, p. 60). Existential questions ask how a person responds in the face of adversity.

Existentialist philosophers long ago noted that the boundaries of human existence are reached in our experiences facing death, suffering, conflict, and fault (Barrett, 1958; Blackham, 1952). These are experiences with which every person must struggle at some point. However, they bring forth not only misery but also nobility, because they refer not only to suffering but also to how one stands against it. The two sides are, in fact, inseparable. As H. J. Blackham (1952, p. 52) put it, a person "may learn to accept them [death, suffering, conflict, fault] as definitive and at the same time find that they are not dead-ends but frontiers where being-in-itself is to be encountered." Each person's life narrative can be mapped across such existential themes.

Existential questions are usually safe to ask because they are normal-izing; they inquire about universal experiences that all humans share and hence require no prior knowledge about a patient's religious tradition. They are reliable because spirituality and religion often stand out among a person's coping strategies for managing adversities. If a person has a meaningful reli-gious life, the conversation turns there after an existential question has been posed. As anthropologist Arthur Kleinman has noted, "Failure and catastro-phe empower religion; religion, in turn, empowers people faced with adversity to overcome self-doubt and fear of failing, and to act in the world" (2006, p. 14). Questions about the impacts of loss or hardship may be empathic, but questions about responses to loss or hardship better reveal a person's resilience (Wade, 1997).

Personal Spirituality Provides Resilience against Demoralization

An existential posture is the readying of one's being—mind, body, and spirit—to respond to adversity (Griffith & Griffith, 1994). As Emmanuel Levinas has noted, "Human moods, such as guilt, fear, anxiety, joy or dread, are no longer considered as mere physiological sensations or psychological emotions, but are now recognized as the ontological ways in which we feel and find our being-in-the-world, our being-there as *Befindlichkeit*" (Kearney, 1984, p. 51). An existential posture describes one's intentional stance toward an anticipated future. For clinical purposes, existential postures can be grouped into those that ready a patient to embrace adversity assertively and those that prepare one for withdrawal or submission.

To guide the crafting of interview questions, existential postures of vul-nerability and resilience can be mapped according to the display in Table 4.1 (Griffith & Gaby, 2005). Existential postures in the left column make up col-lectively the features of demoralization as a human condition. Demoralization refers to the "various degrees of helplessness, hopelessness, confusion, and subjective incompetence" that people feel when sensing that they are failing their own or other's expectations for coping with life's challenges (Frank & Frank, 1991, p. 14). Rather than coping, they struggle to survive. It is apt that "dispirited" is a synonym for demoralization, which feels so much like the disappearance of one's spirit. For many, religion and spirituality serve an important role in buffering or countering demoralization (Griffith & Dsouza, in press).

TABLE 4.1 Existential Postures of Resilience and Vulnerability

Vulnerability	Resilience
Confusion	Coherence
Isolation	Communion
Despair	Hope
Helplessness	Agency
Meaninglessness	Purpose
Indifference	Commitment
Cowardice	Courage
Resentment	Gratitude

[handwritten margin note: Demoralization / disparities]

[handwritten note above table: Coping]

Increasingly, clinical research is investigating the physiological impact of chronic demoralization. Research literature in psychosomatic medicine and psychiatry has associated these existential postures—particularly isolation, despair, and helplessness—with relapse or exacerbation of both medical and psychiatric illnesses (Harris & DeAngelis, 2008; Berkman, Leo-Summers, & Horwitz, 1992; Blazer, 2005; Brown & Harris, 1978; Mookadam & Arthur, 2004; Weihs et al., 2008). They are listed here as existential postures of vulnerability for their roles in both demoralization and the pathophysiology of physical and mental disorders.

The existential postures in the right column of Table 4.1 collectively represent different aspects of assertive coping. Resilience is a capacity to endure hardship or to emerge from adversities in some way stronger than before. In this sense, these existential postures are identified as postures of resilience. Spiritual practices or the practice of a religion help many people to live more of their time within existential postures of resilience (Griffith & Dsouza, in press).

Table 4.1 emphasizes that a person facing adversity simultaneously feels its impact and mobilizes a response, whether to confront or to submit. This list of existential postures is not, of course, exhaustive, nor would these be necessarily the most important for a particular individual's life. One might imagine that "humiliation versus honor," "guilt versus grace," or "contemptuousness versus reverence" might be salient existential themes for different people. Those listed, however, are some that clinicians commonly encounter in patients struggling with illnesses.

[handwritten margin note: a third way - to embrace]

Coherence versus Confusion

Mrs. Richardson was a 75-year-old woman with schizoaffective disorder who also was developing memory problems from Alzheimer's disease. When she told me that she prayed every day, I asked what her prayers were. "I ask God to take away the confusion," she said. "Sometimes, though, I have the nicest thoughts. God hears me sometimes, and sometimes he doesn't. Why do I have so much confusion in my mind?"

Coherence is the capacity to make sense of one's experience.[1] Its counterpart is confusion, as the felt experience of chaos. Coherence is perhaps the most vital of all existential postures of resilience, because confusion largely disables other coping strategies. Before coping can begin, one must be able to discern a pattern.

Confusion in clinical settings can arise from many different sources. Cognitive impairments produce confusion in dementias and during delirium from medical illnesses. They rob a person of the capacity to comprehend one's world. Likewise, the ravages of schizophrenia and dissociative disorders can create confusion for psychiatric patients. Also insidious, however, is confusion that has social origins in our fragmented medical and mental health systems of care. Patients become confused because of missing or inaccurate information from their health care providers or conflicting information arriving from multiple sources. Some questions that help focus on confusion as a problem include:

+ "When in the past have you been able to sort through the confusion and make sense of what you were going through? How did you do that?"
+ "Who in your life most helps you untangle confusing information?"
+ "When you feel confused and uncertain, how do you go about making sense of life?"

---

[1] Ironically, the philosophies of existentialism and postmodernism each help a person to sustain coherence for his or her experiential world by accepting chaos or randomness in the larger world. Existentialism holds tenaciously to a sense of personal coherence by accepting that life as a whole may be random, arbitrary, without implicit meaning. Postmodernism achieves coherency by going even further, accepting that each person is a multiplicity of different selves depending upon whichever dialogue, relationship, or cultural tradition one is immersed in, with no thread running true among them. Despite their ontologies of chaos and randomness, existentialism and postmodernism have thrived since the last half of the 20th century because they have succeeded to varying degrees in helping people to sustain coherency in their personal experiences of living and thus better able to cope assertively.

There are many nonreligious strategies for coping with confusion. However, many individuals, like Mrs. Richardson, turn to their religion when confused, either for the certainty of faith or for a spiritual acceptance of that which cannot be understood. When it is clear that a person follows a religion or spiritual tradition, one can ask more directly:

✦ "When God looks down upon your life, what do you suppose God can see that the people in your life can't fully appreciate?"
✦ "When life feels chaotic, do you have a sense that it somehow makes sense in God's understanding? Do you have any idea what God might understand about your life?"
✦ "Are there ways that your faith helps you manage the confusion?"

Hope versus Despair

"Life doesn't feel worth living," said Ms. Warrenton, a woman in her 60s, after a surgical brain biopsy revealed a malignant tumor. "This has knocked me for a loop. I only have half a brain now," she said, bursting into tears. She was filled with despair, unable to imagine a future.

Hope lies in identifying a desired future and taking steps to build it (Snyder, 2000a, 2000b; Snyder & Taylor, 2000; Weingarten, 2010). Its counterpart, despair, represents resignation and the relinquishing of a desired future (Griffith & Gaby, 2005). Illness often makes it difficult to imagine a future worth living. For patients with medical or psychiatric disorders, despair can pose a greater threat to survival than the disease itself (Harris & DeAngelis, 2008).

Certain questions can open conversations that help patients mobilize hope:

✦ "When did you last feel hopeful? What was that like?"
✦ "Which people in your life most help you to stay hopeful?"
✦ "When times are hard, what keeps hope alive?"
✦ "Who have you known in your life who would not be surprised to see you staying hopeful amidst adversity? What did this person know about you that others may not have known?" (White, 1995)

Such questions often bring forth conversations about religious coping that help sustain hope. Religious faith often is a pillar that supports hope even when life's circumstances leave no statistical probability for good fortune.

Questions about this role for religion, of course, can be asked more directly:

+ "When you feel most discouraged, is there a verse of scripture that brings a sense of hope when you recall it?"
+ "What hope does your spirituality bring to your life that you would not be able to sustain on your own?"
+ "In your religious tradition, what does a person do when feeling overcome with despair?"

Communion versus Isolation

"When you are dealing with more than you can manage, who knows what you are going through? Who notices when things pile up?" I asked Ms. Weldon, a middle-aged woman chronically ill with multiple sclerosis. Her eyes filled with tears, "I'm on duty 24/7 with three children at home. It's just me."

Communion is the felt presence of a trustworthy person. Its counterpart, isolation, is a resigned acceptance that there will be no one there. Medical or psychiatric illness often presses an awareness of who is, or is not, available as a supportive presence (Weihs et al., 2008). Communion differs from "family," "friends," or even "social support." One can, in fact, feel deeply lonely when surrounded by people. Certain questions identify intimate and confiding relationships that count for communion:

+ "When did you last feel the close presence of someone who cares for ⊢ you?"
+ "Who knows what you are going through? To whom do you turn when ⊢ you need help?"
+ "With whom do you feel most comforted when you are hurting?"
+ "In whose presence do you most feel a bodily sense of peace?"
+ "As you go through this illness, how do you stay connected to people ⊢ who matter in your life?"
+ "Toward whom do you most freely express love?" ⊢

Religious, nonmaterial beings—God, saints, ancestors, spirits—can provide a sense of communion for many people. If God's presence can be felt, then one may never feel truly alone. Questions that heighten mindfulness for this kind of communion include:

✦ "Are there times when you feel the presence of God, or is God more like an idea that you think about? At times when you feel God's presence, where in your body do you feel it? What is that like?"

✦ "When you feel God's presence—versus times when you don't feel it so much—how do your symptoms change?"

✦ "When God [your ancestors, your saint] looks upon the situation you are in, what do you suppose God notices most? What might God feel? What might be God's concerns?"

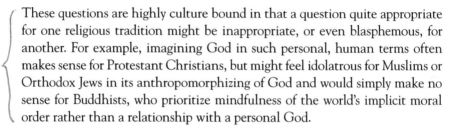

These questions are highly culture bound in that a question quite appropriate for one religious tradition might be inappropriate, or even blasphemous, for another. For example, imagining God in such personal, human terms often makes sense for Protestant Christians, but might feel idolatrous for Muslims or Orthodox Jews in its anthropomorphizing of God and would simply make no sense for Buddhists, who prioritize mindfulness of the world's implicit moral order rather than a relationship with a personal God.

Agency versus Helplessness

Ms. Jones sobbed as she told about the days since her husband suffered a stroke and was left aphasic, unable to understand or to express language. "It's driving me crazy. Nothing I do matters. If I try to talk to him . . . or if I leave him alone . . . or even if I tell him my tears are my fault . . . he still just sits and stares. I can't do this!"

Agency is acting in the expectation that one's actions can make a meaningful difference. Helplessness is acting, or not acting, with an expectation that one's actions make no difference. Often medical and psychiatric illnesses erode a sense of agency. "I had my second heart attack . . . the medical bills were coming in . . . and I couldn't work. It all just piled up."

Reflective questions can be asked that help a person mobilize a sense of agency, following Eric Cassell's maxim that "there is *never* a time when *nothing* can be done" (1991, p. 247). Such questions include:

✦ "When was there a time that you knew you were managing your life well despite this illness?"

✦ "What should I know about you as a person that is not a part of your illness?"

+ "Who helps you to stay strong against this illness?"
+ "How have you managed to keep this illness from taking total control ✳ of your life?"   *be careful here*

When life's circumstances take away any rational hope for control over one's fate, religion locates agency in one's relationship with God or in a divine order. Questions that can heighten this kind of awareness include:

+ "What does God expect of you in a situation such as this?"
+ "Where in this situation might you see the hand of God at work?" ✓
+ "When you pray, do you have a sense that your prayers matter? How?"
+ "What power comes from your spiritual practices and helps you manage difficult situations? What does it enable you to do in this situation that you would not otherwise be able to do?"

Commitment versus Indifference

Mr. Foster became demoralized after his degenerative spine disease resulted in a permanent work disability. "I've always spent my time helping other people," he said. "All my work has been for other people—nonprofits, public service. I've always worked in the government." For Mr. Foster, sustaining morale meant keeping alive the possibility that he could fulfill his sense of purpose, which meant working long hours and contributing service to community projects and nonprofit organizations.

Commitment describes ownership that a person takes for one's life mission, including one's roles, actions, and their consequences. In religious contexts, this has been termed a "calling" or "vocation." Commitment implies not only an awareness that one's actions have consequences for other people, but that certain jobs will not get done, or not get done well, unless one steps forward. The counterpart of commitment is indifference, as detachment from, disregard for, or disavowal of this role and its moral accountability. Some questions that can open discussion of a person's commitment include:

+ "When did you become aware of how your choices affected the other people in your life?"
+ "Who helped you realize how your actions were affecting other people in your life?"

+ "How do you sustain an awareness for how your choices and actions make a difference for others?"
+ "What keeps you from walking off and leaving people to their problems?"
+ "How does your life matter? How does it make a difference that you are alive on the face of the earth?"

For many who are religious, God's purposes stand as the ultimate source from which all individual purposes derive. For some it is an article of faith that God has a specific purpose and plan for each person's life, and one's primary life task is to discern and implement God's plan. Others whose spirituality is grounded in attunement with a moral order also seek to discern one's purpose and to implement that mission. A clinician can inquire more directly about this interplay between commitment and religion or spirituality:

+ "What do you suppose God has in mind for your life?"
+ "For the time left in your life, have you any sense what matters to God that you accomplish?"
+ "Do you ever pray for discernment about your life? From these moments in prayer, what is your best sense of how your life matters?"
+ "During meditation, what are you able to know that gives guidance to how you live each day?"
+ "How do your spiritual practices keep you involved in the lives of other people? Why have you not retreated into your own world and left them to their own devices?"

Gratitude versus Resentment

Mr. Ware, a 25-year-old HIV-positive man became suicidal after learning about his low white blood cell count, which indicated that his viral infection was worsening. "Why me?" he asked repeatedly. He threatened to end his relationship with his partner, who was HIV negative. "He has his whole life ahead of him. I've got nothing. He is going to live. What is the point for me? I've got nothing ahead of me!" he exclaimed bitterly.

Gratitude is an appreciation of desired elements that have occurred among the events and happenings of one's life. Its counterpart, resentment, is the rejection of one's life until certain desired elements appear. Some questions that can help mobilize a sense of gratitude include:

✦ "For what things have you felt most grateful?" ✓
✦ "Despite the sorrow of this illness, for what things do you still feel 🞶 gratitude?"
✦ "Who are the people who have most added something to your life?" ✓
✦ "How do you manage still to feel appreciation for the good things in   – ᴺᴼ – the midst of this much disappointment?"

For many, religion provides a structure of beliefs, practices, and community that facilitates gratitude when the material circumstances of life otherwise would not permit it. When a clinician has a sense for how a person's religion or spirituality matters in life, it can be fruitful to discuss how it bears upon his or her capacity for gratitude:

✦ "Are there ways that your faith helps you to appreciate life even when there is sorrow and disappointment? How does it do that?"
✦ "How does God help you to feel gratitude even on the days when you suffer?"
✦ "Have your spiritual practices helped you learn more about feeling appreciative in your life? How?"
✦ "What are you able to be aware of during meditation that strengthens your appreciation of your life?"

The Timing of Existential Questions

The timing of an existential question during illness or adversity is critical. Asking someone "How do you keep hope alive?" when he or she feels no shred of hope can leave a person feeling unheard and alone. The initial priority is to acknowledge, to listen, and to understand a patient's felt experience, whatever its content. The root derivation of compassion—"to suffer with"—is key in that a patient must first know that a clinician can understand and is willing to feel together the suffering, before opening to the intimacy of such a question as "During the worst of times, from where do you draw hope?" This is the essence of dialogue that Kaethe Weingarten (2003, 2007) has characterized as compassionate witnessing.

Well-placed existential questions often go quickly to the heart of an experience of adversity. Along different planes of a patient's life story, they ask how hardship or loss has impacted a patient's life and how the patient responded. Some patients have drawn more from individual strengths and resources; others have turned more to the strengths and resources of their families, friends, and relational world (Pulleyblank Coffee, 2007; Weingarten, 2007, 2010): "For many this is a hard illness. What gets you through your worst days? What keeps you from giving up? Who understands what you are going through? Who can you count on? What matters most about the days to come?" Because of their universality, existential questions normalize a person's struggle. They ask about challenges that all humans face regardless of power or rank. Stories patients tell are ones of agony, failure, endurance, and triumph. In their fullness, a patient usually comes across as an honorable person doing the best he or she can given the difficult circumstances. Existential questions open conversations about a person's spiritual or religious life in a natural way, particularly when spirituality or religion has previously served a major role in coping.

Situating Clinical Interventions within a Religious Worldview

Even when medical or psychiatric treatment is fully embraced, it is often experienced by a religious patient as only one component within a larger program of healing as defined by religious faith, a 12-step program, or another all-encompassing commitment. When that is the case, clinician and patient can reach a mutual understanding for where professional treatment fits within the patient's religious or spiritual commitment.

For example, Ms. Thompson, a diabetic, suffered from amputation of her left leg and much physical pain from neuropathy. At her internist's urging, she had reluctantly agreed to a psychiatric consultation. At bedside, she was politely dismissive, emphasizing that she was a "born-again Christian."

"Is it your sense that your treatment by Dr. Mallett [her internist] is in accordance with God's plan?" I asked. She said she prayed for Dr. Mallett and felt a sense of peace about his work with her. "Where is the place of this psychiatric consultation in that plan?" I asked. After a pause, she described how much she struggled with despair when her pain was at its peak. We were then able to discuss the use of an antidepressant medication that might buffer the pain while also boosting her energy and sense of well-being. I conveyed my acceptance that her faith was the larger story, and her acceptance of my psychiatric medication was only in support of it.

Such clinical encounters illustrate the sociocultural formulation of a patient's experiential world. Medical anthropologist Arthur Kleinman (1988) has long advocated that clinicians prioritize understanding a patient's explanatory model of illness before proceeding with treatment. Such an understanding can be gained by asking the questions: What do you call this illness? What caused it to happen? How severe do you consider it to be? What kind of treatment do you believe is needed? What do you expect to happen if treatment is given? What do you fear happening? The responses reveal a patient's assumptive world. This assumptive world organizes how a person perceives the world, thinks about it, makes judgments, and acts within it. A clinician is best positioned to provide effective and compassionate care when fully grasping a patient's assumptive world. When counseling a religious patient, asking how a religious perspective informs his or her understanding of the etiology, diagnosis, prognosis, and clinician–patient relationship can play a critical role in understanding that patient's assumptive world. Asking how professional treatment fits within a patient's religious worldview, rather than how religious experience fits within the professional treatment plan, can serve an important role in the sociocultural attunement of clinician to patient.

Questions that help situate medical or psychiatric treatment within a patient's religious worldview include:

+ "Do you feel secure in the medical [or psychiatric] treatment that you are receiving? Do you have a sense whether or not the doctors and nurses are acting in accordance with God's will [or God's work]?"
+ "Do you believe that God has a plan for your life? How do you understand it? How does this treatment fit in that plan?"
+ "How does your spirituality guide you in the care of your health? What spiritual practices do you follow? As you follow the path of your spirituality, where does this treatment fit?"
+ "In addition to psychiatric treatment [or medical treatment or psychotherapy], what else are you doing in your spiritual practices that supports your health and healing?"

Discerning Moral Reasoning within a Patient's Religious Life

Existential questions can help distill personal spirituality out of the muddy blend of family, social, and cultural religiousness. In the process, existential questions also reveal a patient's moral impulses. These moral discernments are often implicit within the patient's metaphors, stories, and beliefs (White, 2007).

Ms. Grant was a 50-year-old woman severely ill with AIDS-related medical complications. For 2 years, she had been sober from the heroin addiction through which she had become HIV infected. During recent weeks, a chronic infection had festered in the tissues of her arm, and her weakened immune system was unable to fight it. Now the blood vessels and nerves in her arm had been so badly damaged that amputation of her arm was recommended. As she weighed this decision, however, she suffered with indecision. Her internist requested psychiatric consultation to provide emotional support.

I asked Ms. Grant how her spirits were holding up through the physical pain and emotional stress of her illness. What sustained her? She nodded, "This is a test." She said that she would willingly bear the severity of the pain if there was a chance her arm would recover. She realized that the surgeons held out no hope and had recommended amputation, but she wavered in accepting their recommendation. She kept asking herself "Is this the right thing to do?" She felt that she had made many bad decisions in the past— with drugs, neglect of her health, and inattention to her additional health needs after HIV infection. Now she felt that her illness had been put upon her as a punishment. From this point on, she wanted to do what was right. She was trying with all her effort. However, she felt that an amputation would be "separating you from a part of your body," and this felt wrong.

"How do you go about deciding what is right?" I asked, "What would tell you that? Who do you talk with about it?"

"It's just something I would feel," she responded, beginning to weep, "but my feelings are all mixed up."

What stood out from this brief encounter was the point of Ms. Grant's concern. It was that she wanted do "what is right" by acting in accordance with her God's wishes. She wanted to put right her relationship with her God. Our conversations sought to understand what her relationship with God required of her. What were God's expectations? With this knowledge as sure footing, she could begin untangling the competing pulls that made her feelings all mixed up: family expectations, church teachings, perceived obligations to follow her doctors' advice.

A right decision is one that lies in accordance with one's values, commitments, and relationships; it does not induce guilt; it will not be later regretted. It requires more than acquiescence to "what I'm expected to do," although obligations to others may carry weight. A decision can be good even though there is nothing good about the situation or the available choices. Moral decision making has not been a primary focus for the mental health disciplines as they have evolved during the past century. Yet making a right decision is a prime concern for many patients facing losses, threats, and uncertainties.

Discerning constituents of personal spirituality orients a clinician to the uniqueness of a patient's moral reasoning and its implications for health and illness. In the Introduction, Ms. Ames initially had made a decision to remain in an abusive marriage because she reasoned, within her religious belief system, that it was the right thing to do. Mr. Chin likewise showed moral reasoning in refusing surgery. It can be important to ask about not only what stresses and challenges a person faces but also how the person reflects upon such questions as, What is the right thing for me to do? What is right for me as a person? What is right for my relationships and commitments?

Informing Sociobiological Religiousness with Moral Reasoning from Personal Spirituality

As personal spirituality is articulated, new meaning can be given to sociobiological aspects of a patient's religious life. Some patients will begin to appreciate how competing strands of religiousness are related to attachment, peer affiliation, social hierarchy, kin recognition, and social exchange. Arthur Kleinman (2006) has used the term "autognosis" for this process of "becoming acutely self-aware of the forces that are shaping us and the directions they are moving us" (p. 231). Wiser decisions can ensue when moral reasoning that is anchored in personal spirituality can be brought to bear upon the sociobiology of religious life.

A general strategy for addressing harmful religion begins by distinguishing personal spirituality from the sociobiological elements of religious life. Asserting the influence of personal spirituality within religious life is the primary objective. Heightened activation of sociobiological processes is deliberately avoided by interacting with patients in a respectful manner that models the compassion and whole-person relatedness that too often have been missing from a patient's religious life. Identifying which sociobiological systems have become most problematic can enable interventions to be tailored to target their specific influences. The weight of clinical intervention, however, falls upon a broad mobilization of personal spirituality and its processes: whole-person relatedness, compassion, existential postures of resilience, generative encounters with the sacred. An emboldened relatedness to persons, not to categories or group identities, is the ultimate aim.

II

✦

WHEN RELIGIOUS LIFE
PROPELS SUFFERING

ATTACHMENT, PEER AFFILIATION, SOCIAL HIERARCHY, KIN
recognition, and social exchange are the "five senses" of social life.
Each of these sociobiological systems extends its sensors into a person's
relational world to monitor how emotions are selected and expressed,
so as to keep strong those relationships and groups upon which a person relies for protection. Much about religious life is a quest for security within relationships—with a personal God; with leaders and peers
of one's religious group; with a host of angels, ancestors, spirits, and
other nonmaterial beings; with churches, mosques, temples, and other
religious organizations. When religious life puts excess emphasis on
strengthen-the-group agendas, however, individual lives of vulnerable
persons can become expendable, neglected, or harmed. A critical area
of discernment for a clinician is whether any aspect of sociobiological
religion so dominates as to override influences of personal spirituality,
with harm for individuals a potential consequence. A clinician's prime
directive is to help a patient reassert the influence of personal spirituality within religious life, balancing religion's valid role for creating
strong social structures with empathy, compassion, and care for self and
others, whether inside or outside one's own religious group.

5

✦

Seeking a Parent in God
Clinical Problems from Insecure Attachments

UNDERSTANDING ATTACHMENT BETWEEN PATIENTS AND THEIR personal Gods provides an emotional vocabulary for making sense out of otherwise inexplicable religiously motivated behaviors. An understanding of attachment theory extends a clinician's skills for grasping the emotional perspective of a patient's relatedness with God. This understanding can be used to anticipate how a patient will respond to life's stresses. It also guides interventions to strengthen the effectiveness of a patient's relationship with God in supporting resilience.

Attachment Relationships

Attachment relationships serve a pivotal role in protecting children by bonding child and parent into an inseparable dyad. Later in life attachment provides the glue that holds together other love relationships. Attachment relationships not only ensure physical safety through proximity to a protector, but they also provide a mechanism throughout life to regulate intense emotions and to sustain the felt memory of intimate relationships. Attachment gives stability to a relational world. Seeking and maintaining contact with another trustworthy and comforting person is perhaps the most profound force throughout human life.

However, attachment can become problematic when its intensity binds people in "stuck" patterns of interaction that generate distress rather than gratification and vulnerability rather than protection (Johnson & Woolley, 2008). Anxious attachments fill life with insecurity and dread. Avoidant attachments produce isolation and loneliness. Either can happen in relationship with one's God as well as in human relationships.

April's Dread of God's Punishing Hand

April was a young woman brought from the hospital emergency room to our psychiatry inpatient unit because of suicidal thoughts and a plan to overdose on medications. She had no history of psychiatric illness or suicidal behavior. However, she had developed panic attacks, nightmares, and fears that "people are going to kill me" after U.S. government agents had forcibly entered her apartment 3 days earlier in search of her Muslim boyfriend. She had been unaware of political activities by her boy friend, who evidently had been under surveillance. April and her mother were handcuffed at gunpoint and interrogated for an hour while their apartment was searched. They were released without charges. Afterward, she reported that "something snapped." Her vigilance was out of control, and she was afraid to fall asleep, remembering that she had been sleeping when the raid occurred. She was admitted to the hospital with a diagnosis of possible acute stress disorder.

The next morning I stopped by April's room to see how she had fared through the night. She was still fearful and tremulous, her story punctuated by sobs. I discussed her symptoms with her, attempting to assure her that, for the most part, she was responding as anyone might after such a frightening event. Then I noticed a note handwritten in pencil on her bedside table:

July 24, 2002

Dear God,

July 23, 2002 changed my life forever. It was the worst day of my life, as you already know. God, they did something to me. In my mind, I keep seeing them. Every day. Every minute. Make it end please. Get those thoughts out of my head.

Your child,
April

I asked April about the letter. I wondered how she hoped God might help and whether she sensed that God had responded. She said that she as a child had observed her Catholic faith but had fallen away from it. She had stopped attending church. She and her mother now argued much of the time. She felt guilty about her relationship with her boyfriend. Now she felt that she had been punished by God.

By the next morning her more severe anxiety symptoms had abated. However, she was still afraid to leave the hospital lest feelings of panic return. There was another letter at her bedside:

July 25, 2002

Dear God,

First and foremost, I would like to apologize to you for all the wrong that I have done. It was only the Devil. What I was doing was wrong, and I knew it. That's why I stopped but it was too late. You had already decided for me to learn the hard way. I learned and I swear on everything I love I will never do those things again. I put my faith and trust in you, Lord, and that you will help me get through this. I need your help. The Devil has made me weak, and I need you in order to be strong, to make me stronger. Keep me from all harms whatsoever. I want to start with a new me, clean and dirt-free. You know what I mean. You see everything.

> *Your child,*
> *April*

Gauging her ambivalence about psychiatry, I felt that she would more fully respond to a chaplain than to a psychiatrist. She agreed with this proposal. I consulted a hospital chaplain, who also was an ordained Catholic priest. He visited April, talked and prayed with her about her relationship with God, and returned the next day to check on her. Feeling her anxiety to be manageable, she asked to be discharged from the hospital by the end of the weekend. She was uncertain about seeking further psychiatric treatment but planned to reestablish her relationship with her church and religious community.

Clinically, April was showing acute anxiety symptoms in the aftermath of a traumatic event, worrisome but possibly still within the range of a normal response from which she might recover uneventfully without psychiatric treatment. From a diagnostic standpoint, her symptoms had not yet persisted long enough to justify diagnosis of a psychiatric disorder. Although she had been given medication to help her sleep, antianxiety and antidepressant medications have not been shown to be of long-term benefit for patients with acute posttraumatic symptoms. Rather, interventions to strengthen coping, educate about symptoms, mobilize social support, and teach skills for de-arousing the body would be more appropriate recommendations. They would help reduce her physiological level of alarm and lessen a longer term risk for posttraumatic stress disorder.

April's religious faith stood out as a core element of her coping. Potentially, it could provide a de-arousing sense of security from God's presence that might help prevent her posttraumatic symptoms from progressing. Yet her letters to God made her religious faith sound more problematic than helpful. Her letters to God displayed an anxious attachment style that risked amplifying her fear and uncertainty instead of relieving it. April felt herself to be weak and unworthy as she approached a God who appeared distant, judging, punishing, and notably lacking in compassion. She worried about her tenuous relationship with God. In frenzied supplication, she sought to regain God's favor, yet her insecurity about the relationship was making it more a source of anxiety than comfort.

I could not know whether this was a reflection of April's long-standing style of relating to her God. Activation of anxious attachment behaviors is a common consequence of acute traumatic stress. Moreover, I was a secular psychiatrist who was positioned poorly as someone who could aid her in sorting through the perplexities of this relationship and her choices within it. The Catholic priest did so more ably.

Joan's Too Far Away God

The case of Joan represents the other end of the religious attachment spectrum. Joan was a middle-aged woman who had made several suicide attempts after a head injury suffered in a motor vehicle accident. Brain injuries left her so cognitively impaired that she was no longer able to work as an accountant. Grief over her inability to read and to do math seemed unending. She told me, "You do reading, writing, and arithmetic all the time and never think about it. You never know what words mean until you can't read anymore." She was certain that she did not desire life if this was what it meant.

I knew that Joan had attended church regularly before the accident. I asked her where she experienced God in her situation. She said she had always believed that God knows everything that will happen in each person's life from the moment of the person's birth, which meant that her suffering must have been in some way planned by God or had some purpose in God's eyes. She described God as now "like an old man, far away," a creator perhaps but not a being to whom one would turn for comfort. She could not imagine God feeling compassion for her, but feared God's judgment if she were to commit suicide.

Although Joan expected little from God, she still felt guilty that "I haven't put God number one in my life." She wondered whether God had given up on her because of her doubts. When she contemplated suicide, she asked, "Why is it that it doesn't matter what Bill and Janet [husband and daughter] think, but it matters to me what God thinks?" She wished to feel free of God so that she could feel free to die.

Joan related to her God with a dismissive-avoidant attachment style. She only trusted her own capabilities. She felt that God might hold power in the universe but was disinterested and unavailable to her. God was not a being who could be counted on. God would not be a source of comfort for her suffering.

What stood out with both April and Joan was that their beliefs *about* God were less the issue than their emotional experiences of relationship *with* God. They each encountered limits as to what were the felt possibilities of the relationship.

Understanding Person–God Interactions through the Lens of Attachment

Attachment researchers have made distinctions between an attachment relationship and a person's attachment style. A person has, at most, only a handful of attachment relationships. These are the primary parenting figures or caretakers during the first years of life, which point to a lifelong bonding to parental figures that humans share with other mammals. The emotional contours of attachment relationships, however, also set more general expectations about worthiness of self and reliability of others when interacting in future relationships. These generalized expectations, or attachment styles, become a legacy of one's early life relationships that continue throughout life to shape each new love or friend relationship. Empirical research studies have found that attachment relationships are permanent fixtures throughout the life span. Attachment styles appear to be more malleable during adult life. A person can learn to become self-aware about one's particular attachment style, placing it in context rather than giving it sole play when interacting with people. A person can learn new ways of relating that are superimposed on the old, thus changing the outcomes. Even though insecure attachments do not disappear, there can be hope that insecurely attached adults can learn how to live beyond their limits, even when their influences are still felt.

Attachment styles broadly shape the relational worlds within which people live. Insecure attachment styles explain why some patients with factitious disorders produce fabricated illnesses and self-injurious acts—swallowing sharp objects, taking surreptitious overdoses of medications, falsifying laboratory data to appear ill—in order to feel secure under the watchful caretaking of a doctor. They explain why other patients, emotionally unable to tolerate feelings of trust, refuse to adhere to their treatment regimens despite the serious nature of their illness (e.g., diabetes, epilepsy) and awareness that treatment noncompliance could result in illness, disability, or death (Stuart & Noyes, 1999; Ciechanowski, Katon, Russo, & Walker, 2001). Like Bill Murray's character in the film comedy *What About Bob?*, a patient with an anxious attachment style may generate symptoms of illness, even fabricating them, in order to keep close proximity to a caregiver. Like Emile Hirsch's portrayal of Christopher McCandless in the tragic *Into the Wild*, a patient with an avoidant attachment style may sabotage or flee therapeutic relationships repeatedly lest feelings of dependency or intimacy emerge.

Attachment styles carry over from human beings to divine beings. They provide a clinically useful paradigm for understanding the otherwise puzzling array of ways that people relate to their personal Gods. Thus, a secure attachment style can mean that a person is able to sustain felt assurance that God is present and responsive when needed. Because God will be available, there is no reason to be anxious. By contrast, a person with an anxious attachment style may believe God to be strong and capable but feels uncertain that God will be available. Such a person may feel too weak or unworthy to merit God's attention. Religious life, therefore, becomes preoccupied with entreating, placating, or otherwise worrying about God's availability, attachment behaviors reflecting a low threshold for activation. A person with an avoidant attachment style falls at the other end of the spectrum, with attachment behaviors activated only by extreme conditions. Avoidant attachment styles can be subtyped as dismissive or fearful. With a dismissive-avoidant style, the person feels God to be emotionally distant, either disinterested or unable to assist in times of need. Such a person expects little from God and relies only upon oneself. With a fearful-avoidant style, the person feels closeness with God to be too unsettling and hence avoids God and relies only upon one's self (Kirkpatrick, 2005). People with attachment problems fare no better with God than with any other relationships.

Interestingly, one's attachment style is a factor that strongly influences the probabilities for a religious conversion experience. Most people with dramatic religious conversions have anxious attachment styles, and a smaller number have avoidant attachment styles. People with secure attachments to God tend to have religious lives that actively influence daily behavior, but with few religiously dramatic moments. Although the suddenness and intensity of behavioral change during conversion can be striking, people with anxious attachment styles ironically also are more prone to forsake their religious commitment at later points in time (Kirkpatrick, 2005).

Awareness of a patient's attachment style can provide a way to make sense of emotionally intense interactions with one's God that otherwise might appear nonsensical. Attachment describes how a human being utilizes, or does not utilize, the felt presence of this parent-like relationship with God to feel secure when frightened, uncertain, or overwhelmed. It describes how people under stress seek out or veer away from God as a source of comfort. Awareness of a medically or psychiatrically ill person's attachment style with God can go a long distance in explaining why his or her interactions with God can, at times, be perversely maladaptive.

Insecure Attachment: No Shelter from the Storm

Assessing attachment style between a patient and his or her God can help a clinician find empathy for a patient's suffering. It can also guide the tailoring of clinical interventions. Ms. Johnson in the Introduction can be contrasted with either April or Joan described earlier in this chapter. Alone in the hospital, in pain, healing slowly from surgical wounds, burdened by layers of concerns about children at home, Ms. Johnson still found consolation in the felt presence of her God: "By his stripes I am healed." She did not think she could have endured the stress of her illness without God to rely upon. Like Ms. Johnson, a patient securely attached to his or her God can turn to this relationship for comfort and security when facing illness, disability, or death. Secure dependence upon one's God also enables a more coherent and positive sense of self. For many, one of the Bible's most beloved passages is Psalm 23: "Though I walk through the valley of the shadow of death, I will fear no evil for Thou art with me." These verses speak the emotional truth about a relationship with one's God, not simply a declaration of religious ideology. Someone who senses such assurance generally feels no need to prove its validity, and someone who lacks it has difficulty finding it from theological arguments or logical proofs.

An insecure attachment with one's God often means that a sense of comfort and security is not obtained from the felt presence of God. When attachment is insecure, a person is more vulnerable to states of alarm and less able to terminate them by relying upon that relationship. Separation quickly leads to despair and then detachment. An anxious attachment style swings back and forth between angry efforts to coerce closeness and obsessive pursuit of reassurance. An avoidant attachment style fails to activate any relationship-seeking behaviors (Johnson & Woolley, 2008). Either anxious or avoidant attachment styles can be evident in patients' God relationships.

Insecure attachments tend to consume most of a person's attention and are exhausting. Preoccupation with an insecure relationship with God can lead to neglect of self or other human relationships. For example, Ms. Finn was an elderly patient disabled by arthritis. She lived alone, seemingly little attended to by her children. When a family meeting was held, however, a more complex family story emerged. Ms. Finn's two adult children told how their mother had been worried about her salvation as a Christian for as long as they could remember, filling her daily life with religious devotions and study of scriptures. When they were young, they both had obediently attended church, read daily from the Bible, and followed their mother's faith. Their experience of it though had been emotionally empty and joyless. As they grew into adulthood, each had stopped any formal religious practices. They avoided spending time with their mother in part because of their aversion to her religiosity. In recollecting their family history, they both resented the role of religion in their family life, not only for what seemed to them to have been its failed promises but also for how it had taken their mother from them. Ms. Finn's insecure attachment with her God had generated so much anxiety that it became an obstacle to intimacy with her children. The relational stance toward God cost her relationships with her children.

Insecure attachments tend to exacerbate stress-induced illnesses. Analogous to what our government in 2001 seemed to have intended with its Homeland Security "Code Red" terrorist alerts, insecure attachments keep the brain's alarm systems in a state of chronic activation. This overuse, however, produces wear and tear in the body's physiological systems, a process termed allostatic loading. Whether insecure attachment to God can play a specific role in psychosomatic illness is a question that has never been examined in a well-designed research study. Clinical anecdotes, though, are suggestive, as seen in the case of Ms. Panelli, whose constant presence in her primary care physician's office eventually led to a psychiatric consultation. Ms. Panelli's life was poignantly sad. She was a first-generation Eastern European immigrant with no children or close friends. Desperate for human warmth, she clung to a disinterested husband who showed little else but disgust toward her. However, this same pattern of interaction seemed to characterize her relationship with her God. Hours spent with prayers and spiritual practices still left her with uncertainty whether God was near or far away. The results of her worship hardly seemed better than her husband's arid distance. Headaches, dizziness, and fatigue took her instead to her physician, who, in turn, wanted to refer her away to a psychiatrist.

The risks from insecure attachments are greatest when demoralization from adversity provokes suicidal impulses or when humiliation from injustice stirs feelings of revenge. Rather than providing solace or a sense of justice from God's presence, an insecure attachment can instead exacerbate agitation or propel a desperate flight toward God that ends in death. Mr. Miller was a middle-aged man found unconscious, covered in blood, in a grove near the Lincoln Memorial in Washington, DC by National Park Rangers. He was near death following a suicide attempt. Years before a stroke had left Mr. Miller with memory impairment and other cognitive disabilities. He lost his job and then his marriage. He now lived at a subsistence level on Social Security disability checks. Surgeons in the emergency room resuscitated him and sutured his wounds. As I admitted him to our psychiatry unit, he told me, "My only hope lies in the promises and salvation of God." He had cut deep lacerations in each of his arms and legs, then across his throat, in a desperate effort to join God in heaven.

Assessing Person–God Attachment Style

In practical terms, there are three types of attachment styles that concern clinicians: secure, anxious, and avoidant. It can be useful to subdivide the avoidant category into a fearful-avoidant attachment style, in which a person keeps distance from God because of a fear of retribution, and a dismissive-avoidant attachment style, in which a person feels that God is unreliable and not to be counted upon. Psychologist Lee Kirkpatrick (2005, p. 110) has provided a succinct summary of person–God attachment relationships in terms of the relative regard given self or other during interactions. It is based on the cognitive framework that organizes the attachment style. Table 5.1 summarizes key distinctions among the different attachment styles.

Attachment theory is sometimes mistaken for a cognitive theory, as though attachment styles were no more than beliefs or ideas. For example, I once was chagrined to receive as a comment in a review of a manuscript submitted for publication: "The author refers to God as an attachment figure and later refers to attachment theory as a way to understand one's link to God. This betrays a problem with the paper and psychiatry. The author needs to help the trainees to understand how believers think about their God. It is certainly not through attachment theory that this will happen." This comment reflected a naïve, but common, perspective. The popular psychology of our culture often assumes optimistically that people can change their relatedness with others in a straightforward way through education or by adopting more enlightened beliefs. This may be true for certain kinds of relational problems. However, it

TABLE 5.1. Attachment Styles toward a Personal God

Attachment style	Emotional quality of personal relationship with God	Associated beliefs about God
Secure	"God feels close, loving, and compassionate toward me."	"God is a being who is loving and reliably present."
Anxious	"I feel unworthy of God's love."	"God is a loving being, but his love for me is conditional or unreliable."
Dismissive avoidant	"I feel that I can rely only upon myself."	"God is a distant and unreliable being—a relationship with God counts for little."
Fearful avoidant	"I feel unworthy of God's love, and I fear God may punish me."	"God is a distant being who can be threatening."

is often the case that relational problems are not amenable to efforts simply to change how one thinks. People with major problems from insecure attachments find themselves imprisoned by the limits of their emotional relatedness. In her psychoanalytic studies, Ana-Maria Rizzuto described patients who were atheists yet who could not stop feeling tormented by a God they no longer believed existed (Rizzuto, 1979). A more common problem is that a patient professes strong beliefs that a loving God exists, yet is emotionally unable to feel closeness with that God or to take comfort in the relationship. These kinds of problems bear the stigmata of insecure attachment and often are not remedied by simple reassurance or changing theological beliefs.

Clinicians who accurately assess a patient's attachment style with his or her God can better gauge what are reasonable expectations for that patient–God relationship as a source of comfort and security for a distressed patient. Awareness of attachment style opens a door to empathy with patients whose ways of relating might otherwise be off-putting. A problematic insecure attachment with God can serve as an appropriate focus of psychotherapy, sometimes using trustworthy human relationships as a bridge to a more trustworthy relationship with one's God (Griffith & Griffith, 2002).

Person–God Attachments in Psychotherapy

Problems involving insecure attachments with one's God often do not present similar obstacles to engagement in psychotherapy as problems embedded in other sociobiological systems. Problems involving sociobiological systems of social hierarchy, peer affiliation, kin recognition, and social exchange are primarily about group behaviors. Attachment is about a private, dyadic, emotional relationship with one's God. An insecure attachment with one's God does not necessarily build a rigid boundary around religious identity that keeps a secular clinician at a distance. Problems of insecure attachment, in fact, often lend themselves well to the methods and techniques of psychotherapy. ✓

Insecure attachments with God can be addressed in psychotherapy in a similar manner to interpersonal problems in other couple or dyadic relationships. In the Introduction, Ms. Dylan's fearful-avoidant attachment style with her God kept her alone and bereft at the very point she most needed solace and comfort from God as she coped with disabling multiple sclerosis. Her psychotherapist was able to work with her dyadic relationship with God in much the same manner that one would address any other conflicted couple or family relationship.

An attachment perspective tends to inform psychotherapy in either of two ways. First, as a tool of empathy, accurately assessing an attachment style toward God helps a clinician to anticipate the realistic limits to which a patient may be able to utilize God as an emotionally supportive relationship. Such an assessment can help a clinician feel compassion for a patient's plight when a God whose existence is affirmed by religious beliefs nevertheless provides surprisingly little comfort or solace in practice. Second, as a goal for therapeutic outcome, the course of psychotherapy can shift when it is appreciated that God, in fact, serves a key role within a patient's relational world. For example, Karl found his way to me for couples therapy after asking colleagues for a referral to a psychotherapist who might take his Catholic faith seriously. Karl's childhood and adolescence had been turbulent years: fighting with parents, abusing alcohol and marijuana, and pursuing love relationships that repeatedly moved through a cycle from intense passion to boredom to abrupt endings. During college Karl converted to Catholicism in order "to devote my whole life to God, to leave the chaos I have lived in since the day I was born." After briefly considering the priesthood as a vocation, he instead chose to marry. Karl waited to propose marriage, however, until his priest had met his girlfriend and communicated his favor upon their union. Now, 2 years later and with a newborn child, Karl still felt a lingering yearning to become a priest or monk who could devote all his waking hours to prayer and the worship of God. It was only during ecstatic prayer that he felt his anxiety disappear and "a relaxation deep in my gut." He described a dream in which "God's face was close. I felt brilliant yet calm, and wanted to shout, 'God is everywhere!' I felt awed by this." The problem that brought Karl and his wife to therapy was that he could not find a similar passion and deep comfort in his relationship with her. Once articulated, however, the openness, comfort, and ecstasy of this relationship with God did provide for Karl an awareness of what could be possible in the intimacy of a relationship, a beacon that could guide him in other relationships. He committed himself to working in couple therapy to find this openness and wonder in his marriage.

Leveraging Human Relatedness to Change Insecure Attachment with God

When an insecure attachment with God appears unworkable, it sometimes is possible to use a human relationship as a secure base from which the insecure person–God relationship can be addressed. Joan, the accountant whose avoidant attachment to God was presented earlier, experienced a progressively worsening depression and multiple suicide attempts in the 2 years after her motor vehicle accident. Medications for anxiety and depression only partially buffered her distress. She could make only limited use of psychotherapy because her concentration, memory, and capacity to think abstractly were so limited. After yet another serious suicide attempt, her frustrated husband left her.

Several months later, Joan came for an appointment looking unexpectedly content. She told how she could feel gratitude now for the first time in years and was glad to be alive. After her divorce, she felt as empty as a tomb. Yet she remembered words that her grandmother once told her as a little girl: "Prayer changes things." She decided to go with her parents to their small rural church. After the first visit, she felt nothing, became angry, and refused to return for a month. However, she eventually returned and joined an adult Sunday School class, where she met Roger, who was also divorced. Roger was a thoughtful, gentle man. They became close friends. He was interested in the small moments of her day and her accomplishments as she struggled with tasks of daily living. She felt comfortable talking with him, unembarrassed about her obvious neurological impairments.

In time Joan and Roger married. Joan's transformation was remarkable. She began venturing into stores alone to shop, showing no shame for mistakes made attempting to write checks or trying to remember what items she came to buy. For the first time in the 4 years I had known her, she was willing to attend family and social gatherings where her aphasic errors using language had previously brought unbearable humiliation.

Notably, however, Joan also talked about a transformation in her relationship with God; something had happened spontaneously shortly after she married Roger. She began feeling God's presence. She no longer felt deeply alone. Whereas she had once characterized prayer as "empty as praying to those pine trees outside the window," she now felt comforted by God. With other family and church members, she began helping some of the poorer families in the community. "There's been a lot of prayers answered," she said. "It feels good to be back in church. I didn't realize how important it was."

Joan was able to use secure human relationships to bring life to her stale ⟵ and empty relationship with her God. First, her relationship with her dead grandmother, then her relationship with Roger, brought her into a new state of being in which she could trust and receive comfort from her God. Her neuropsychiatric symptoms had fluctuated little over this interval. Although psychotherapy, family therapy, and a complex psychopharmacological regimen had partially ameliorated her mood and cognitive symptoms, their benefits had been limited. There was little else to which the steps she began taking toward her God plausibly could be attributed.

Deconstructing a Fearful-Avoidant Attachment to God

Lydia was a patient who coped with many illnesses: inflammatory bowel disease and arthritis, in addition to chronic posttraumatic symptoms from abuse in childhood. She was treated in a chronic pain program with high doses of a narcotic, which added to her isolation because she could not drive safely with the medications.

Lydia admonished herself harshly for becoming a disabled person. I was concerned about the impact of this self-punishment on her low morale. I challenged this but received from her only a shrug of acknowledgment: "Well, what do you expect?"

One day I posed it differently. "There are circumstances—your injured joints, your gastrointestinal symptoms—that neither you nor I know how to change. But I'm concerned that you have a surplus of suffering from your self-judgments that I believe is not obligatory. When in your life did you learn to N8 measure yourself against tough standards?"

"It's my Presbyterian upbringing," she responded.

"What do you mean?" I asked.

"I'm supposed to pray that I get better," she added.

"Do you have a sense that God hears your prayers?" I asked.

"Not any more," she answered.

"Once you did, but not now?" I asked to clarify.

She nodded, weeping.

"What sense do you make of that?" I asked.

"I don't. I feel I'm being punished," she responded.

"Do you have the sense that God hears other people's prayers?" I asked.

"Yes. I'm sure he hears my parents' prayers," she answered.

"Why not yours?" I wondered.

"I don't know. You know there are people who do very bad things but nothing bad happens to them," she said with resignation.

"Yet you feel you are being punished?" I finished her sentence.

"I believe that," she answered.

The avoidant quality of Lydia's attachment style with her God was evident. It brought no strengthening or solace, but only added to the weight of her illness. I challenged her to grapple with it. My hope was that we could lessen its contribution to her suffering.

"You have so much to cope with," I responded. "Your body has as much as it can manage with these illnesses. It is not good for it to have the added burden of the negative emotions—blame, shame, guilt—from these judgments upon yourself. You already have enough to handle. It's not fair. Can we talk a bit about where in your life you learned how to tell the difference between what is reasonable and not reasonable to expect of yourself?"

The focus of discussion shifted to Lydia's childhood growing up in a family with parents and siblings who were high achievers, while she struggled with a chronic physical illness that curtailed her education and opportunities for professional accomplishments. Her self-perceptions of unworthiness were sealed when she was sexually assaulted as a teenager, leaving her with long-standing posttraumatic symptoms. They infiltrated her religious experience, cohering into a sense of herself as a person bypassed by God's love for inexplicable reasons. This deconstructive inquiry repositioned the focus of psychotherapy, making evident the nonreligious origins of so much of her guilt and opening the question of what may have been missed from her religious life from her presumption of God's condemnation.

The Role of Attachments to God within Religious Sociobiology

Nearly 30 years ago, I stumbled unexpectedly upon God as an attachment figure in my psychotherapies with religious patients. Like many, I had assumed that a person's religious beliefs also indicated the quality of emotional relationship between that person and his or her God. That is, I expected a person whose theological beliefs emphasized God's compassion and inclusive concern for humankind to have a warm, heart-to-heart relationship with a God characterized by love and acceptance. I likewise expected that a person whose theological beliefs emphasized moral judgment and punishment for sins to have an austere relationship with an angry God or a God of stern expectations. Although some of my patients did show this congruence, many did not. Some fundamentalist individuals worshipped a "fire-and-brimstone," God of judgment in their theology, yet described an intimate personal relationship with a God who was compassionate and understanding even through times of moral failure. Others experienced a personal God who was harsh and judgmental, even though their liberal theology espoused a God who gave love and acceptance freely to all humankind. Still others with liberal theologies lived daily lives of remarkable commitment and compassion, yet described a personal God who sounded detached and mechanistic. It seemed ironic that this God seemed to have much to learn from those who worshipped him. My assumption that one's religious beliefs also predicted one's quality of related-ness with God was quite wrong. Much more was going on.

Sigmund Freud, in fact, had grasped this a nearly 100 years earlier. From his psychoanalytic data, Freud considered the "God imago"—the emotional image of God within consciousness—to be a part of primary process cognition and related to internalized emotional images of one's parents (Rizzuto, 1979). He considered religious beliefs, however, to represent secondary process cognition, an overlay of rational thought superimposed upon, and often not well connected to, the deep currents of primary process thinking. Subsequently, psychoanalytic scholars such as Ana-Maria Rizzuto (1979), William Meissner (1984), and John McDargh (1983) furthered the study of God as an intrapersonal reality. Rizzuto regarded the God imago as "the last internalization" that occurred after the Oedipal period and added God to the pantheon of parents, grandparents, and other early caregivers whose felt presences would be reckoned with throughout one's life (Rizzuto, 1979). The object relations psychology within which Rizzuto articulated her work was in many ways a forerunner of attachment theory and gave similar guidance to clinical work.

Attachments with God are a major component of religious sociobiology, yet they are not the whole story. God as an attachment figure is most evident within the private conversations and interactions that a person has with God, rarely witnessed by others. Attachment relationships with God have relatively little to do with religious identities lived out in the social behaviors of religious groups. To count as an attachment relationship, a relationship with God must meet the criteria of proximity, safe harbor, and secure base. God must be felt to be potentially available in times of distress if the attachment is secure or deliberately or incompetently unavailable when the attachment is insecure.

Many positive (and negative) relationships are governed by processes other than those of attachment (Kirkpatrick, 2005). A member of the Unification Church may have a passionate, idealizing relationship to Reverend Moon as leader of the Church. However, this may better fit a social hierarchy paradigm rather than attachment, to the extent that the church member has no expectation that Reverend Moon will be physically available during a moment of need (Kirkpatrick, 2005).

Here an analogy to particle physics may be apt. Four forces, the strong and weak nuclear forces, electromagnetism, and gravity, appear to hold the universe together (Griffiths, 1987). Although gravity is the force that we witness all around us, from apples that fall from trees to the movements of stars in galaxies, it has only a minor role in keeping the matter of the universe glued together. The strong nuclear force is 10 billion times stronger than gravity but only operates at a distance of one-billionth of a meter. The strong nuclear force holds together the protons of atoms. Gravity is so weak, by contrast, that it would seem to be negligible, yet it becomes the only force that we daily witness because it operates across distances of millions of miles. Gravity holds together galaxies. An attachment relationship with a personal God is like the strong nuclear force, giving a hard stability to religious experience at the most elemental level, yet unseen in the rich pageantry of religious organizations, public worship, doctrinal beliefs, and other religious social life that we most commonly think about as religion.

In a psychotherapy that is focused on the interior life of a person, attachment to a personal God becomes prominently visible, and its essential role in critical life decisions is obvious. God as an attachment figure often does not follow the tracks laid down by a one's logically reasoned beliefs about God. A God attachment has more the ambivalent character of a relationship with one's parents, vital in importance yet often feared or resented as well as loved. Attachments to God often churn anguish and darkness, not just sweetness and light.

6

Seeking Security within the Flock
Clinical Problems from Social Hierarchy, Peer Affiliation, and Reciprocal Altruism

PERHAPS NO FORCE IN THE HUMAN WORLD IS SO POWERFUL AS the attachment between a parent and child. It is sobering then when religion's influence so completely overrides this bond that a watching parent makes no effort to intervene as a child suffers and dies, or the parent even becomes complicit in the death. Such occurrences speak to sociobiological processes in religious life whose scope extends beyond the intense, but dyadic, bond of attachment.

In spring 2008, the corpse of Javon Thompson, a toddler, was discovered in a Philadelphia shed packed into a suitcase stuffed with mothballs. Detectives identified Javon's mother as a member of One Mind Ministries, an offshoot Christian religious sect in Baltimore. Upon learning that 16-month-old Javon had stopped saying "amen" at mealtimes, the group's spiritual leader, Queen Antoinette, had determined that the boy had a demonic spirit that needed to be cleansed through fasting. She ordered that he be denied food and water until he repented. Javon's mother watched over him as his skin darkened with dehydration. Slowly, he fell quiet and died. Group members placed Javon's body on a mattress in a back room and prayed for days that he would be resurrected from the dead. They eventually concluded that the resurrection ritual failed because someone within the group did not have sufficient faith (Morse, 2009).

Javon's mother had always shown an affectionate relationship with her son. There was no history of her abusing him. Court-appointed psychiatrists found her to have no diagnosable mental illness in that her individual beliefs were indistinguishable from those shared with others in her religious group.

The macabre account of Javon's death and failed resurrection was disturbing for an additional reason. Arrested for murder, Javon's mother resisted separation from the religious group or blaming it for the death of her son. A year earlier, her family had tried to persuade her to leave the group. Forbidden by the group leader from visiting her grandson, the grandmother remembered hugging her emotionless daughter on the sidewalk outside the One Mind Ministries building. "It was like she was a complete stranger," she recalled.

A more elaborate account of a child's tragic death from a family's religious practice is the memoir of the Parker family, *We Let Our Son Die* (Parker, 1980), which also has been produced as a movie, *Promised a Miracle* (Weisberg & Clark, n.d.). Larry and Alice Parker and their 11-year-old son, Wesley, centered their family life in their local church, where they gathered with friends for worship and Bible study (Griffith & Griffith, 2002, pp. 215–218). Wesley suffered from insulin-dependent diabetes. A traveling evangelist preached a religious revival at their church, claiming the healing of his physical disability by faith. The evangelist assured church members that they also could be healed from illnesses if they placed their faith in God. During a prayer, Wesley felt the touch of God's hand. He believed he had been healed. Encouraged by the prayers and fervor of family and friends, Wesley threw away his insulin, needles, and glucose-monitoring equipment. Over tortuous days and hours, Wesley slowly sank into coma and then died, as his parents stood by him (Parker, 1980).

Unlike Javon's mother, who lived in a marginal religious cult, the Parker parents were typical middle-class citizens attending an unremarkable Protestant Christian church. It was obvious that neither the parents, Wesley, their fellow church members, nor even the evangelist was mentally ill. All had strong religious faiths and the best of intentions. Yet the human drama in which they each participated was madness. Religion can produce madness when no one involved in it is, in fact, mad.

These stories from our day call to mind the ancient tale of Abraham and Isaac on Mt. Moriah. Abraham, spiritual father of Jews, Muslims, and Christians, abandoned his eldest son, Ishmael, to the wilderness and then years later prepared to sacrifice his remaining son, Isaac, on Mt. Moriah because he perceived God to require this of him (Genesis 22: 1-24). Isaac's near-slaying has since preoccupied 2,500 years of Jewish, Muslim, and Christian scholarship in efforts to understand or explain away Abraham's nonresistance to filicide. It even helped launch 20th-century existential philosophy through Soren Kierkegaard's 1968 study of Abraham's actions in *Fear and Trembling.* An angel stayed Abraham's hand and spared Isaac. No angel stayed the deaths that befell Javon and Wesley.

Seeking a Model of Religion That Explains Religious Harm

A clinical approach to counter harmful uses of religion must rest upon a comprehensive understanding of religious life that includes within its scope both the protection it provided during Ms. Johnson's illness (presented in the Introduction) and the vulnerability to harm produced in Javon's and Wesley's deaths, explaining both out of the same set of ideas and concepts. It must explain not only how religion can at times prescribe harmful behaviors but also the failure by others present to challenge the harmful acts. An adequate understanding of harmful religion thus must answer three questions:

1. How does religion prescribe harmful behaviors?
2. What inhibits protest by participants and witnesses?
3. How do some religious people become actively complicit in committing harmful acts?

A strategy for answering these questions shows how social hierarchy, peer affiliation, and social exchange systems motivate behaviors designed to strengthen the integrity of a religious group. At times, however, these group-focused behaviors can harm vulnerable individuals within the group or outsiders who do not belong to the group. Influences of these sociobiological systems act both externally and internally to choreograph group members' conduct. Externally, they selectively reinforce behaviors of high value for group integrity. Internally, they alter how an individual group member processes attentional and emotional streams of information, thereby reconstituting his or her sense of self. Activation of social emotions—pride, honor, embarrassment, shame, guilt, humiliation, and the like—provides continuous online monitoring of individuals' behaviors, keeping them closely aligned with group agendas. Such monitoring produces within individuals a virtual "sociobiological self" that stays closely attuned to group expectations. Emergence of this sociobiological self necessitates dissociative suppression of incongruent aspects of a personal self, which involves silencing an individual's spontaneous thoughts, feelings, and actions. An individual's moral reasoning loses its voice.

This chapter explicates how these sociobiological systems and the subjective worlds of religious individuals interact. Chapters 7 and 8 then return to the hospital bedside and psychotherapy office to show how this conceptual framework can guide clinical work.

Social Hierarchy, Peer Affiliation, and Social Exchange Provide a Social Cytoskeleton for Religious Life

Social hierarchy, peer affiliation, and processes of social exchange build a social cytoskeleton in religious groups that offers members a robust structure for their lives. These sociobiological systems did not originate as religious phenomena. They evolved to meet the practical needs of early hunters and gatherers for survival. Now, however, they organize religious life along similar lines as were the social priorities of hunters and gatherers. On a positive side, these sociobiological systems enhance efficiency and effectiveness of religious groups in their strivings to survive and grow, which can hold secondary benefits for group members. The confluence of these sociobiological systems ensures a sense of security, often powerfully so. Collectively, they contribute to the "relief effect" that new members often feel when first joining a cohesive religious group (Galanter, 1999). They uplift morale for individuals by lessening any sense of isolation, providing a group purpose in which each individual can share and endowing a sense of power through joint effort.

Yet each sociobiological system in its own way can place an individual at risk for harm when needs of the individual cross purposes with what best serves security for the group. The sociobiological systems in their influences can expand to encompass most of religious life. Then a sense of self as an individual can wither and, with it, processes of personal spirituality. A panoply of suffering can emerge for those involved when religious life is reduced only to its sociobiological elements.

Social Hierarchy

Social hierarchy dictates an uneven distribution of power in groups so that some have more access to resources than others, and some do more of the work than others. This is as true of religious groups as secular ones. Hierarchies of power seem unavoidable. They emerge spontaneously in nearly all animal species from crickets (Dawkins, 1989) and crayfish (Barinaga, 1996) to chimpanzees (Boehm, 1999), indicating their evolutionary importance. Although size, strength, and sexual attractiveness determine social status in most species, social power effected through alliances and coalitions becomes more important among higher primates, such as chimpanzees and humans.

Humans live in social systems largely organized by language, where dominance is more often achieved through verbal intimidation and seductive rhetoric than by physical violence. Prestige plays a major role. Prestige refers to status that is conferred by lower status group members who hope to benefit from the leader's skills, abilities, or knowledge. Prestigious individuals are revered rather than feared (Kirkpatrick, 2005). Everyday religious life is largely constituted by interactions around power and status, dominance and submission, prestige and subservience as members of churches, synagogues, mosques, and temples interact with each other, their religious leaders, and the supernatural beings they worship.

Religious social hierarchies are most often organized around the perceived supreme power of God. In religious social systems, God's role is commonly that of a family patriarch or imperial ruler: "our Father in heaven," "ruler of all," "mighty Lord." Charismatic religious leaders have well-honed skills for assuming stand-in roles for God, which accrue a similar king-like status. In the company of their followers, God and human religious leaders activate sociobiological systems for dominance and submission much as do leader dogs with their packs, lions with their prides, and alpha males with their primate troops. Hardy (1966) drew a direct parallel between human relatedness with their Gods and "canine devotion" to their human masters, attributing the close bonding of dogs to humans to a combination of a prolonged maternal attachment and dominance behavior. Although many intimate interactions between a person and his or her God can be regarded as processes of attachment, the placating and submissive displays that commonly characterize public worship—bowing, praising, pleading—better fit the dominance and submission processes of social hierarchy (Kirkpatrick, 2005).

Social hierarchy evidently must form if a religious group is to endure successfully with an impact upon its society. Victor Turner (1969) described how efforts to sustain group communitas—social encounters in which people relate to each other in emotional fullness without regard for status or rank—inevitably devolve into social structures with hierarchy, roles, and functional relationships, because practical work must get done. The communitas of a utopian community, a religious revival, a political movement, or the early days of Orwell's *Animal Farm* may be emotionally exhilarating, ethically righteous, and aesthetically appealing, yet ineffective in completing work necessary for the group to realize its competitive goals.

Although necessary and inevitable, religious social hierarchy often values obedience and submission in ways that open a door to exploitation, abuse, and self-neglect. Karen Armstrong in *The Spiral Staircase* (2004) described the sequelae of her 7 years as a Roman Catholic nun. She entered the convent as an idealistic but naïve 17-year-old intent upon a spiritual quest, an epic adventure, to live in "the infinite and ultimately satisfying mystery that we call God." This did not happen. In her words, "I entered in 1962 as an ardent, idealistic, untidy, unrealistic, and immature teenager, and left seven years later, having suffered a mild breakdown, obscurely broken and damaged" (p xi). She spent the ensuing decades seeking to rebuild an intellectual and emotional life from the wreckage. What went wrong in Karen Armstrong's spiritual journey centered on the primacy of "the rule" in her religious order. She later recalled the stringent punctuality required of the novitiates:

> At the first sound of the convent bell announcing the next meal or a period of meditation in the chapel, we had to lay down our work immediately, stopping a conversation in the middle of a word or leaving the sentence we were writing half written. The rule which governed our lives down to the smallest detail taught us that the bell should be regarded as the voice of God, calling each one of us to a fresh encounter, no matter how trivial or menial the task in hand. Each moment of our day was therefore a sacrament, because it was ordained by the religious order, which was in turn sanctioned by the church, the Body of Christ on earth. So for years it had become second nature for me to jump to attention whenever the bell tolled, because it really was tolling for me. If I obeyed the rule of punctuality, I kept telling myself, one day I would develop an interior attitude of waiting permanently on God, perpetually conscious of his loving presence. But that had never happened to me. (p. 3)

 What began as a search for the open, free, spontaneous presence of God became transformed into a submissive lifestyle in which thoughts and actions, at levels of minute detail, were specified and prescribed. Experiencing the presence of God was redefined in terms of rules, roles, and acts of self-censorship. These proved not to serve Armstrong well as she searched for a felt presence of God. For her religious order and church, though, these were time-proven methods for making young nuns pliable for their service.

Peer Affiliation

Affiliative bonds between people who initially are strangers can strengthen to family-like intensity in religious groups where individuals share in common religious idioms, beliefs, and practices. Activation of kin selection mechanisms has been put forward as the most parsimonious explanation for member-of-the-pack behaviors in religious groups (Kirkpatrick, 2005). Peer affiliation is about loyalty that group members commit to one another. Semper fidelis, the U.S. Marine motto, is sometimes unofficially translated as "always faithful—unit, country, God, in that order."

Kin selection is generally regarded as one of the core processes that have driven human evolution. Recognizing, supporting, and furthering the well-being of one's blood kin is a straightforward mechanism for advancing the reproductive success of one's genes. That kin selection should operate to huddle bloodkin into clans of mutual protection against outsiders is not surprising. What is more intriguing is how language and social practices, rather than blood, can be used to cement similar clans made up of nonkin individuals. Groups that are bonded tightly around political ideology, totemism, or shared language can in fact approximate the affiliative intensity of bloodkin. Crippen and Machalek (1989, p. 74) have proposed that a cognitive sleight of hand can be used so that "kin recognition mechanisms are 'usurped' to form communities of fictive kin." Kirkpatrick (2005, p. 249) has described as "kin-talk" the ways that religious groups use the language of "our heavenly father" (implying a common familial ancestry) and "brother" and "sister" (implying shared filial relationships) to co-opt social processes that originally discriminated only purely biological markers, such as smells or body shapes. Kin recognition and peer affiliation can mutually potentiate their effects to create religious groups that powerfully suppress the behaviors of individual members that deviate from the religious group identity.

Jerome Groopman (2004), looking back across a long career as an oncologist, wrote *The Anatomy of Hope* to teach what he had learned over the years about helping patients with cancer to sustain hope. In his last year of medical school, he recalled Esther, a 29-year-old Jewish woman who had been diagnosed with breast cancer. When he examined her, it was obvious from the size of the tumor and nearby lymph nodes that she must have been aware of the tumor for years but had not sought medical attention. As she lay in a recovery bed after her mastectomy surgery, she startled Groopman, her assigned medical student, by confiding to him a secret: "My cancer is a punishment from God." She explained that she had consented to a sexual relationship with her boss. It had served as a window to the world outside a suffocating marriage that had been arranged by her parents. In short, private conversations, Esther said enough for Groopman to grasp her plight. It was clear how nothing could be revealed to her family, rabbi, or community without the risk of extrusion and shunning. "I carry it with myself, alone," she said. "Markus [her husband] talks to the rabbi, my mother talks to God. I can't talk to either." Groopman realized that she lived in a world of family and community role expectations in which she felt invisible as a person and helpless to protest any aspect of her existence. He too knew no way to help her with her dilemma. She refused chemotherapy and quietly died.

Social Exchange and Reciprocal Altruism

Altruistic behavior within social groups occurs through social exchange processes in which group members act in ways that benefit other group members without prioritizing regard for self. If all group members abide by principles of reciprocal altruism, the group can gain a powerful evolutionary advantage. As a strategy for group survival, "all for one and one for all" holds a competitive edge over every group member narrowly pursuing self-interests. Basketball teams and military platoons prevail to the extent that they can foster a culture of reciprocal altruism within their group. Evolutionary psychology has put forward substantial evidence that reciprocal altruism is not simply trial-and-error learning but is based upon hardwired mammalian systems that are easily activated in group settings (Gintis, Bowles, Boyd, & Fehr, 2003; Singer et al., 2006).

Social exchange with God and other supernatural beings is a dominant theme in most religions. Usually a religious person assumes that an understanding about social exchange exists with God. In ancient religions, crops, animals, and even children were sacrificed to God. If God's favor could be incurred, then crops would flourish, cows would give more milk, and hens would lay more eggs. The idea of the tithe in Mosaic teaching was a giving back to God one-tenth of one's possessions, with the idea that God in time would reward the gift.

Reciprocal altruism is typically embedded within religious beliefs that promote group cohesion and the longevity of relationships between group members. Pargament (1997) has detailed the myriad ways in which a person's church, synagogue, temple, or mosque serves as a social network of material and emotional support. Throughout the world, a Christian, Muslim, Jew, or Hindu generally can step into a place of worship and find community regardless of age, gender, or ethnicity. Few other social institutions or other kinds of organizations can make a similar claim.

At the most abstract level, social exchange and reciprocal altruism have given us our ethical standards of conduct and notions of justice. Morality has been widely regarded as an evolutionary product of mechanisms designed to promote reciprocal altruism (Alexander, 1987; Ridley, 1996; Kirkpatrick, 2005). Kirkpatrick (2005) has noted that certain basic moral precepts for reciprocal altruism, fair social exchange, and detection and punishment of cheaters are nearly universal across the world. Thus, Rabbi Hillel the Elder declared for Jews (Armstrong, 1993, p. 72): "Do not do unto others as you would not have done unto you." Christians similarly follow Jesus's admonition: "Do unto others as you would have others do unto you" (Armstrong, 1993, p. 81). A Hindu aphorism is: "Do not to others what you do not wish done to yourself; and wish for others too what you desire to have done unto you; and reject for others what you would reject for yourselves." In Islam, it is: "Do to all men as you would wish to have done unto you and reject for others what you would reject for yourselves." In Confucianism: "Do not to others what you do not want done to yourself" (Peterson, 1986, pp. 74–75). Fair social exchange is embedded deeply and universally within the human psyche. ARGU

A sense of a "just world" in which good is rewarded and evil punished appears to be a product of our evolved social exchange systems. Most people carry a sense that justice is implicit in the world. This expectation is explicitly stated by the Buddhist and Hindu Law of Karma and in the talion justice of "an eye for an eye, and a tooth for a tooth."

However, there is a dark side to expectations of reciprocal altruism with ✓ humans and fair social exchange with God. People can irrationally accept bad fortune as God's punishments for personal sins, as did Ms. Dylan in the Introduction or April in Chapter 5. A person also can overstay a role or a relationship in which he or she is exploited in the expectation that such sacrifice will be rewarded eventually. A person can even commit self-execution when feeling that one has committed a violation for which no just punishment was served. The plot of the 1980 Academy Award-winning film *Ordinary People* turned on such an event. The story opens with a suicide attempt by a high school student, Conrad. As the story unfolds, a psychotherapist, Dr. Berger, pieces together the story: Conrad and his older brother were sailing on a lake when a storm upended their sailboat. Conrad stayed with the floating boat keel, as sailors are instructed to do; his brother though swam for shore and drowned. The film has been a popular one for psychotherapy seminars because there are multiple psychological formulations that can be put forward to explain the connection between the drowning and the attempted suicide. One of these, however, is a moral interpretation: that Conrad tried to kill himself because he believed it was the right thing to do: Justice served meant that he too must die as did his brother. Survivor guilt can be lethal.

There also are more subtle ways in which expectations of fair social exchange foster exploitation in families and social groups. In the Biblical story of Jacob and Esau, Jacob fled into the wilderness after manipulating his father, Isaac, to bestow upon him the family birthright, which ought to have gone to his older brother, Esau. In the desert country of Medea, Jacob, in turn, found himself used and manipulated. He fell in love with Rebecca, his employer's daughter, so struck a deal with her father, Laban, that he would tend the flocks and herds 7 years in return for her hand. Then Jacob found the tables turned on him by tribal birth-order law. At the end of 7 years, Laban explained that tradition required that the eldest daughter, Leah, not her younger sister, Rebecca, be first wed. Jacob persisted. He grudgingly agreed to marry Leah then work an additional 7 years to receive Rebecca as well, followed by yet another 7 years to receive sufficient animals and servants in payment, as his household with two wives and children would require for self-sufficiency. After 21 years, though, Jacob did receive his due (Genesis 28–29).

The problem with the Jacob story is that it communicates a message that faith and good works will in the end be rewarded even if much delayed by greed, dishonesty, and misdeeds of others. For many the payoff never comes, and the Jacob story and similar moral tales only serve the rhetorical interests of unscrupulous politicians and businessmen whose intentions from the start are to exploit to the greatest extent possible and for as long as it can last. This was an aspect of Western Christianity that Friedrich Nietzsche so scorned as a herd mentality (Barrett, 1958).

How Can Religion Prescribe Harmful Behaviors?

The shaping of religious life by sociobiological systems opens a straightforward path through which harm can come to individuals. In daily life, sociobiological processes of social hierarchy, peer affiliation, and social exchange usually operate collectively as an ensemble. They act to internalize social norms and expectations, as such becoming editors of self-expression. These internalized social norms and expectations place parameters upon a person's perceptions, feelings, and actions to align them with group priorities, whether or not these priorities converge with needs of the individual. The end product is a newly fabricated self, a sociobiological self, tailored to fit social roles and obligations. A person acting out of this sociobiological self prioritizes group expectations above competing individual needs of self or others.

Untoward Effects from the Sociobiological Editing of Religious Life

Suppression of individual desires can be used by groups to amplify commitment to the group. Javon's mother and Wesley's parents each were put to a test, asked by their spiritual leaders to embrace religious beliefs and practices that defined their group religiousness but by putting their children at risk for harm. In each case, their turning away from normal parental instincts bolstered the perceived power of group bonds.

Psychiatry and psychology for 100 years have struggled to understand how such internalization happens, in which social processes restructure an individual's psyche, orienting it to act on behalf of social roles and expectations rather than self-interests. In the 1920s, Lev Vygotsky (1986) described internalization from a Marxist perspective as a normal process of intrapersonal development, in which cultural forms and social practices configure a child's inner speech and thought to the point that the child begins reproducing the cultural forms and social practices spontaneously and autonomously. According to Vygotsky, that which is subjective and intrapersonal always begins first in the interpersonal social world around the child.

At the same time, English psychoanalysts were describing internalization from their psychoanalytic perspectives. Melanie Klein, an early object relations psychologist, posited that emotional images of parents invaded a child's psyche, which they continued to inhabit as quasi-parasites, making trouble throughout the child's life. Psychoanalyst D. W. Winnicott (1965) produced a more sophisticated version of object relations psychology, proposing that a child aesthetically creates a "false self" to suit the expectations of family and society, while protectively hiding away a "true self" that is a private repository of personal thoughts and spontaneous feelings. Winnicott felt that the task of psychoanalysis was to discover the true self and to help a patient to take vigorous and public ownership of it.

Social philosopher Michel Foucault (1973, 1980) described internalization differently as a tool of social power. Foucault documented the movement of Western societies since the Enlightenment toward training citizens to think about their lives in terms of normalizing judgments that measured their own and others' behaviors against scientific and professionally prescribed standards. Those who disciplined themselves to think and act consistently within these specifications soon started self-monitoring themselves without the watchful eye of an external authority. The prescribed standards were then internalized.

Vygotsky, Winnicott, and Foucault each pointed to a human capacity, perhaps universal, for creating multiple autonomous selves, each operating as independent centers of reasoning. One self has been consistently identified by its attunement to role and relationship expectations from family, group, and society. The other has been shown to be a source of spontaneous thoughts, feelings, and impulses belonging to the individual.

What sociobiology adds is an explanation for why this is necessarily so. From a sociobiological perspective, power is effected by inclusion or exclusion from social groups, by social structures that limit access to resources, and by relational rules of dominance and submission. The formation of a sociobiological self ensures that an individual can stay on the winning side of groups who wield power.

Long before Facebook or MySpace, people have created sociobiological selves as "false selves" for social networking purposes. Most humans do so with little mental effort or internal dissonance. This suggests that the human nervous system has been designed so that a part-self can step in as a whole self when interacting with others. An often unacknowledged mission for parental religious instruction and parochial teaching—Sunday Schools, Jewish day schools, madrasahs, public worship services—is to hone children's sociobiological selves for smooth participation in future public and organized forms of religion.

By contrast, personal spirituality only operates through participation of one's whole being. Personal spirituality grows and develops within the province of personal self—Winnicott's territory of the "true self." Its agendas are directed toward the welfare of oneself and other persons in their individualities, not toward expectations of religious social structures and power hierarchies. Problems in religious life appear when sociobiological self and personal self collide in their strivings.

What Inhibits Protests by Those Who Witness Religiously Driven Acts of Harm?

Social emotions—embarrassment, shame, guilt, humiliation, pride, honor, admiration, and others—are the guardians of human sociobiology. Within the brain, social information and emotional information are interactively processed in order to manufacture socially adaptive behavior. Relationships and emotional expression are carefully coregulated (Norris & Cacioppo, 2007). Social emotions promote compliant behavior by preoccupying attention with how one is perceived by others. When strongly felt, little attention is left for responding to inner stirrings of one's personal self. Social emotions enforce the editing of religious behavior by a sociobiological self, to such an extent that protests are inhibited even as harm happens.

Personal spirituality requires a capacity to act in accordance with spontaneous and unedited empathic and compassionate emotional responses. It is about listening for small movements of one's human heart. The influence of personal spirituality is expectedly weak when religious life is largely about pride, honor, shame, humiliation, or guilt. Sometimes social emotions have been referred to as prosocial emotions, following the argument that all people would be sociopaths in their absence and societies could not exist, hence their evolutionary importance (Gintis et al., 2003). However, they are prosocial *sic !* only in the sense of equating prosocial with group success, a definition that could have been embraced by Stalinist Russia.

Sociobiologically, the social emotions differ in the roles they each typically serve. For example, pride, honor, and admiration motivate people to achieve culturally mandated standards of excellence (Norris & Cacioppo, 2007). Embarrassment propels a person to "fix oneself" by attending more carefully to social norms and expectations. Shame is more intense than embarrassment: It readies a person to hide, to camouflage, to avoid being witnessed by scrutinizing and judging gazes of others. The archetypal image of shame in the Western world is Adam and Eve in the Garden of Eden, in full flight while frantically covering themselves with grape leaves in order not to feel the eyes of God burning upon their skin. Guilt, by contrast, is an emotion that motivates a person to make restitution or to repair injury done to another. Whereas shame is about perceived defects in oneself as a person, guilt is about wrongful acts (Lazare, 1999, 2004). Humiliation is emotional aggression. A humiliating act forcibly lowers the other in social status, pain that is magnified by the presence of real or imagined witnesses. Humiliation feels to be a violation, hence the quickness with which it mobilizes resentment, bitterness, and retaliation. Acts of humiliation are never forgotten and move quickly to physical violence, as in duels of honor or blood feuds (Lazare, 1999, 2004; Malcolm, 1998, pp. 19–20).

Social Emotions Suppress Public Expression of a Personal Self

Each social emotion subjugates self-awareness and expression of spontaneous feelings to the force of social expectations. Social emotions provide moment-to-moment modulation of social interactions. They keep people behaving *argu* within bounds of group roles, attending to responsibilities, and submitting to leadership and hierarchy. The Talmud teaches "to shame someone is to shed their blood" (Lazare, 1999). The social emotions powerfully shape the daily lives of people. They are the social glue of groups and communities. In religious life, however, their suppression of individual expression can exact great costs. These costs can include the disappearance of those, like Esther, who cannot find a space within their bounds where life feels worth living.

How Do Some Become Complicit
in Religiously Driven Acts of Harm?

Sociobiological systems can do far more than simply edit overt social behavior. They also can reach deeply into the minds and hearts of individuals, altering how they subjectively experience their lives as they notice, desire, and think. Religious social structures, internalized heavy-handedly by social emotions, result in the highly edited, sometimes constricted, normative behaviors that observant religious persons often show in public settings. However, this is insufficient to explain the emotional flatness and robot-like vacuousness often witnessed among members of cults and to varying degrees in other cohesive religious groups.

When religion acts destructively, those involved often act more as accomplices than as victims under duress. Cult members liberated from abusive religious leaders by their families often defend the actions of the leader, even seeking to return to the cult (Singer, 1995). Religious fundamentalists search their sacred scriptures to justify violence toward those outside their groups, building logical arguments why hatred, coercion, or even murder is godly. Self-inflicted suffering is reframed as joy.

Why this should happen might seem puzzling. After all, politicians, actors, business leaders, and professional consultants of all sorts show masterful internalization of role behaviors and a nuanced responsiveness to social emotions. Yet such professionals usually show animated personalities with vigorous personal agency and autonomy alongside their sociobiological selves. Performances of social role behaviors can be turned on and off. Julia, in George Orwell's *Nineteen Eighty-Four*, is an iconic figure as a secret rebel within a totalitarian state, where she publicly led praises for the ideological doctrines and rule of Big Brother (Orwell, 1949). Privately, she lived a bohemian, ruleless life that spoke her contempt for Big Brother's mores. She took pride in how fluidly she could move between the two. Few Julias are to be found among the religious in settings such as Jonestown, the Heaven's Gate Cult, or fundamentalist churches where spousal or child abuse is blessed through justifications from sacred scriptures.

Dissociative Silencing of Personal Moral Sensibility

Personal spirituality is largely an awareness of spontaneous moral impulses felt while attuning emotionally and attending fully to another person or oneself. Breakdowns in attunement or lapses in attention can disrupt guidance by personal spirituality.

Cohesive, tightly structured religious groups can call upon their individual members to put aside plans for a career or marriage, to silence complaints about personal losses and humiliations, to show public affection for other group members who act repugnantly, to toil endlessly without compensation. Ethnographic accounts of religious cults provide numerous such examples (Galanter, 1999; Singer, 1995). Karen Armstrong's story provides poignant illustrations for each of these points within one of the world's mainstream religions. There often is no voiced protest from a personal self as individual sensibilities are dampened. This silencing of personal self operates unseen within individuals. Volitional choices can play a role, as when one deliberately engages in "biting my tongue" or "swallowing feelings." It can also happen involuntarily, without volition, as when "I just got caught up" or "it just seemed natural."

Emergence of a sociobiological self appears to be no more than half the formula for placing religion at high risk for destructive ends. The other half is an active suppression of personal moral sensibility by processes that are internal to individuals. As a sociobiological self ascends in prominence, a capacity for emotional awareness and attentiveness to self or others steadily disappears for many members of cults and religious groups. Vitality of personal spirituality dissipates with it.

The Neurobiology of Dissociative Self-Silencing

Dissociative processes are the strongest candidates as psychological mechanisms for suppressing personal moral sensibility. Dissociation refers to mental operations that compartmentalize and separate different regions of experience, including a capacity to split away feelings that ordinarily would accompany perceptions (Maldonado & Spiegel, 2008a). Mental processes become separated so that they seem to occur independently.

A capacity for reabsorption of personal self into a mode of being defined by sociobiological specifications may be a universal legacy of our evolutionary past. The first-person experience of this has been articulated by philosopher Martin Heidegger (1962), who noted how one's being-in-the-world already has been defined before a child becomes self-aware, even before birth. Heidegger's insight is summarized by William Barrett (1958, pp. 219–220) as follows:

> We are each simply one among many; a name among the names of our schoolfellows, our fellow citizens, our community. This everyday public quality of our existence Heidegger calls "the One." The One is the impersonal and public creature whom each of us is even before he is an I, a real I. One has such-and-such a position in life, one is expected to behave in

such-and-such a manner, one does this, one does not do that, etc., etc. We exist thus in a state of "fallen-ness" (Verfallenheit), according to Heidegger, in the sense that we are as yet below the level of existence to which it is possible for us to rise. So long as we remain in the womb of this externalized and public existence, we are spared the terror of the dignity of becoming a Self. . . . Because it is less fearful to be "the One" than to be a Self, the modern world has wonderfully multiplied all the devices of self-evasion.

Heidegger observed that an individual Self that had emerged during the developmental years of childhood often becomes reabsorbed later to varying degrees back into a mode of public existence, because this is less fearful. This tension stands in the background of awareness, which is why the most fundamental of moods is anxiety (angst) as an intuitive awareness of "this here-and-now of our existence [that] arises before us in all its precarious and porous contingency" (Barrett, 1958, p. 221). From a neurobiological perspective, systems within the human brain that enable this hibernation of self may have been hardwired from the beginning.

Brain processes involved in dissociation have been shrouded in mystery ever since Pierre Janet's theories of the 1800s. Dissociative processes have both voluntary, conscious, explicit components and involuntary, unconscious, implicit components. Many dissociative processes are normal and common occurrences during daily life, including daydreaming, performing tasks automatically while attention is preoccupied and failing to notice pain when distracted elsewhere. There are psychopathological forms of dissociation that constitute mental illnesses, with the boundary between normal and psychopathological still controversial (Spiegel, 2008; Maldonado & Spiegel, 2008a). Over the past decade, however, advances in brain electrophysiology and functional brain imaging are finally explicating how dissociative processes may operate within the brain and within a person's social interactions. Clues for how dissociative self-silencing might operate come both from laboratory studies of normal dissociation and studies of dissociative phenomena in psychiatric disorders.

Hypnosis: A Model for Normal Processes of Dissociation

Hypnosis is a form of normal dissociation that has provided a useful experimental paradigm for studying dissociative self-silencing in the research laboratory. Hypnosis research has studied how normal dissociative processes can be mobilized to alter a person's perception of reality. As such, it may help us understand how religious group processes can produce disappearance of an agentic, self-reflective self.

Hypnosis is a psychophysiological state in which a person shows attentive absorption, a range of dissociative phenomena such as perceptual and memory distortions, and a high level of suggestibility (Maldonado & Spiegel, 2008b). When hypnotized, a person shows complete immersion in a central focus of attention while inattentive to all else in the background. Hypnotists throughout the ages have been surrounded by dark tales about their powers for placing people in robotic trances in which a person follows an authoritarian master's commands automatically and without questioning. However, it is now appreciated that "all hypnosis is self-hypnosis" (Maldonado & Spiegel, 2008b, p. 1986), in that the role of a hypnotist resembles more that of a coach or mentor than a dictator (Kihlstrom, 2008). Hypnosis requires a series of assents from a subject that create an expectation of followership toward the hypnotist. Consequently, skilled hypnotists, like telemarketers and politicians, have a bag of rhetorical tricks that seek to establish this "yes-set," so people can be lulled into docility. Once a hypnotic trance is established, a subject still holds the power to act in opposition to the hypnotist, but when in a trance state of mind the thought of resisting just does not come up as something to think about.

Most people are hypnotizable to some degree, and about one-fourth of adults markedly so (Hilgard & Hilgard, 1983). Highly hypnotizable individuals can conduct complex behavioral tasks while amnestic, can experience parts of their bodies as numb, can feel time speeded up or slowed down, or can be blinded selectively to the presence of certain physical objects but not others (Erickson, 1980; Erickson & Erickson, 1980; Barnier & Nash, 2008). Most children are highly hypnotizable, with a peak for hypnotizability occurring between ages 8 and 12, which then slowly declines until adulthood (Hilgard & Hilgard, 1983). High hypnotizability is a correlate of intense religious experiences (McClenon, 1997).

Neurophysiological research studies have suggested in rough outline how the brain produces hypnotic alterations in conscious awareness (Barabasz & Barabasz, 2008; Fan, McCandliss, Sommer, Raz, & Posner, 2002; Spiegel, 2008; Posner & Peterson, 1990). In hypnosis, the brain's executive systems of the prefrontal cortex work in concert with its major distributor of attentional resources, the anterior cingulate gyrus, to inhibit selectively neural circuits elsewhere in the brain. This produces states of consciousness in which one or more sectors of sensation, motor function, or self-awareness are omitted (Hofbauer, Rainville, Duncan, & Bushnell, 2001; Spiegel, 2008; Maldonado

& Spiegel, 2008b). Omission of these sectors permits an experiential reality to be constructed based on partial awareness.

That hypnotic dissociative processes are so universally distributed among human beings suggests their evolutionary importance. They provide a way in which focused attention can disengage the experiencing self from sources of suffering in the environment. On the whole, it seems merciful for humans to have a capacity for hypnosis.

The hold of hypnotic dissociation on awareness appears never to be complete, however. There always seems to exist what hypnosis researchers have termed the "hidden observer" (Hilgard & Hilgard, 1983, pp. 166–169). This refers to a remarkable human capacity for a subject in a hypnotic trance to respond to questions as if specific sensory, motor, or memory functions were fully disabled, yet with a "hidden observer" simultaneously aware of the performance, as if watching the whole scene like a fly on the wall. Even though a subject with a hypnotically anesthetized arm may deny feeling any pain when the arm is submerged in a bucket of ice water, a hypnotist can then address the subject's hidden observer, who accurately gauges the severity of pain. Moreover, hypnosis cannot obliterate the autonomic changes in pulse and blood pressure that accompany the physical pain, indicating that the pain is "really" felt even when denied. Conscious awareness of this dissociative self-silencing is thus partial, fluctuating, with some gradation of liminal awareness that it is happening, as in "at some level I probably knew," "I just pushed it off to the side," or "I think I just didn't want to know."

Hypnotic procedures and dissociative experiences of daily life connect human beings with the rest of the animal kingdom. The capacity for dissociation may be built into the central nervous system of every human being, with some people—the highly hypnotizable—more gifted at it than others. Hypnosis has provided a neurological mechanism for limiting suffering even when physical sensations of pain are still felt (Rainville, Duncan, Price, Carrier, & Bushnell, 1997; Rainville, Hofbauer, Bushnell, Duncan, & Price, 1999; Rainville, Hofbauer, Bushnell, Duncan, & Price, 2002; Price, Barrell, & Rainville, 2002). An analogue of dissociation, the immobility reflex or freeze response, sometimes termed "animal hypnosis," exists in other mammals, reptiles, and amphibians as a survival mechanism that is triggered by extreme threat (Gilman & Marcuse, 1949; Klemm, 2001).

Depersonalization: A Model for Pathological Dissociation

Hypnosis as normal dissociation can be compared with pathological dissociative states that occur as a symptom of major psychiatric disorders. In pathological dissociation, there occur profound distortions of one's sense of self or of one's body (depersonalization), altered perception of space or time (derealization), automatic behaviors occurring outside awareness (fugue), disabled memory processes (psychogenic amnesia), or hallucinated images, sounds, or body sensations (Simeon & Abugel, 2006; Maldonado & Spiegel, 2008a). In severe forms of pathological dissociation, such as dissociative identity disorder, there is little semblance of a coherent self that can be sustained across different moods and states of mind. Pathological dissociation occurs commonly among individuals who have experienced emotional neglect or abuse over a prolonged period of time, particularly if this occurred during the childhood years of personality formation (Maldonado & Spiegel, 2008a).

Depersonalization disorder is a milder dissociative disorder that might bear some semblance to the vacuousness seen among members of religious cults. Depersonalization disorder is rarely so disabling that a person cannot function in daily life (Simeon & Abugel, 2006; Holmes et al., 2005). A person with depersonalization disorder generally sustains a clear sense of self despite suffering that can ensue from specific symptoms. People with depersonalization disorder often experience feelings of unreality and disappearance of one's sense of self. There are feelings of detachment and emotional emptiness or flatness. Daily life can have a disconcerting "as if" sense, as though one were observing oneself from the outside or viewing oneself acting a role in a movie, much akin to the hidden observer of hypnosis. Concentration is difficult, and one's sense of time or hearing, seeing, and touching the physical world may feel distorted (Simeon & Abugel, 2006). Jean Paul Sartre's (1938/1962) portrayal of Roquentin, his protagonist of *Nausea*, grasping the root of a chestnut tree, unable to feel aware of it or to recollect words for it, while "alone in front of this black, knotty mass," has stood as one of literature's most vivid portrayals of depersonalization. People with depersonalization disorder feel unreal much of the time, too aware of thoughts, feeling hollow, and emotionally disconnected (Simeon & Abugel, 2006).

Social practices that induce depersonalization also bear resemblances to the induction procedures of cults. Psychologists James Cattell and Jane Cattell identified the emergence of corporate cultures and institutional bureaucracies of the post-World War II era as sources of increasing depersonalization within American society: "People working under centralized bureaucracies are routinized, humiliated, and thereby dehumanized. The economic system prevents involvement and fosters detachment" (Cattell & Cattell, 1974, p. 768). Cattell and Cattell (1974) showed how social practices of standardization were impacting the way individuals experienced themselves as persons. They argued that bureaucracies and corporations entrain workers into a kind of docility in which awareness of personal self atrophies. As a specific illustration, Hochschild (1983) conducted an ethnographic study of the training of Delta Airlines flight attendants. Hochschild showed how symptoms of depersonalization were a by-product of corporate efforts to train flight attendants to suppress not only outward expressions but even private awareness of negative feelings when dealing with irritable, rude, or hostile customers.

Depersonalization disorder shares with the anxiety disorders a capacity to rob life of its richness, while preoccupying the sufferer with constant awareness that one's mind is malfunctioning. Religious cult members often show an emotional flattening and detachment resembling depersonalization disorder. If hypnosis provides a laboratory model for dissociative self-silencing in religious groups, depersonalization disorder may provide a psychopathological model.

Simeon and Abugel (2006, pp. 105–125) have reviewed evidence for how depersonalization operates neurobiologically. In depersonalization disorder, two abnormal brain processes are suggested by drug studies and functional brain imaging. First, heightened activation of the medial prefrontal cortex and anterior cingulate gyrus, as in hypnosis, suppresses the amygdala and hippocampus, which are the gateways through which sensory information enters the limbic system and where emotional responses are to be generated. Second, the sensory association cortex of the parietal lobe, particularly the right angular gyrus, fails to activate normally. The right side of the brain ordinarily provides an embodied awareness of self, as discussed in Chapter 2. Right-hemisphere processes are anchored in direct awareness of the state of one's body and its emotional state. Normally, self is distinguished from other by comparing left- and right-hemisphere activations (Decety & Grezes, 2006; Lamm et al., 2007). For example, it has been known that the angular gyrus region of the right parietal lobe is a sensitive area where epileptic discharges produce out-of-body experiences, and strokes can produce loss of awareness that the opposite half of one's body even exists (Devinsky et al., 1989; Mesulam, 2000, pp. 218–219). Neurobiologically, a person with depersonalization disorder preserves a sense of self but lives with a brain whose capacity to feel the emotional valence of sensations is dulled, and systems fail to integrate information arriving from multiple sensory channels into a full-formed image of one's embodied existence.

Patients with depersonalization disorder are often highly hypnotizable, suggesting that hypnotizability might be a factor predisposing to depersonalization (Simeon & Abugel, 2006). The same brain circuits may be involved in both. Whether or not religious depersonalization bears any direct relationship to hypnosis or depersonalization disorder, the kinship of certain symptoms such as emotional emptiness, detachment, and constricted sense of self among members of cults and cohesive, ideologically driven religious groups suggest shared circuitry for information processing.

An Integrated Model for Dissociative Self-Silencing in Religious Life

When the findings of clinical psychiatry and social psychology are joined with neurobiological research on hypnosis and depersonalization, a model takes shape that can help explain how dissociative suppression of personal moral sensibility may occur routinely in cults and other cohesive religious and ideological groups.

Emergence of a personal self within the sociobiological constraints of families and family-like social groups is always a tenuous negotiation. Both provide benefits: Families and social groups provide physical and emotional security, while emergence of a personal self brings cognitive and emotional autonomy that can be used to care for self specifically as an individual. The optimal balance between the two depends on what future is regarded as the best prospect.

Neurobiologically, the prefrontal cortex is the likely arbiter of negotiations between sociobiological and personal self. It fixes its course upon an envisioned future that could be worth living. Depending upon its estimation of possibilities for this future, the prefrontal cortex can activate or deactivate sensorimotor systems elsewhere in the brain or adjust subcortical systems that govern movement away from or toward sources of threat or gratification.

The human brain is above all a social brain. The sociobiological systems heavily bias the prefrontal cortex to attend to attachment, peer affiliation, social hierarchy, kin recognition, and social exchange considerations in setting its course. When security and support for morale are most needed, full sway is thus given the sociobiological systems. The prefrontal cortex, in conjunction with dorsal cingulate systems, can close off access from the outside world to the feeling-generating limbic system. Parietal lobe systems for distinguishing self from other can be taken offline, so that self-awareness and spontaneous expressions of personally felt emotions disappear. Such a person operates in partial shutdown mode, with only the sociobiological self standing as self. Consequences of this partly dehumanized but functional state can become ominous in the broader expanse of life.

Legacies of Dissociative Self-Silencing:
Bad Faith, Doubling, Unspeakable Dilemmas,
and Their Human Costs

Dissociative processes appear to play regular roles in harmful acts that are justified by religious beliefs or ideology. Multiple efforts have been made to explain how this can happen. In part, these explanations differ in how they apportion responsibility to conscious or unconscious choices, although each affords some role to both.

After surviving Auschwitz, Primo Levi (1988) spent the remainder of his life producing a factual account of how those in the death camp—killers, victims, bystander witnesses—responded to its demands. He described how they perceived, thought, and felt as well as actions they chose. In *The Drowned and the Saved*, Levi (1988) distinguished between those who told deliberate lies to hide their complicity in the genocide and those who learned to hide lies from their own awareness. He described a particular type of self-deception as a common coping mechanism through which perpetrators and complicitors sought to regain entry to civilized society. Levi (1988, p. 27) observed:

> Under such conditions there are it is true those who lie consciously, coldly falsifying reality itself, but more numerous are those who weigh anchor, move off, momentarily or forever, from genuine memories, and fabricate for themselves a convenient reality. The past is a burden to them; they feel repugnance for things done or suffered and tend to replace them with others. The substitution may begin in full awareness, with an invented scenario, mendacious, restored, but less painful than the real one; they repeat the description to others but also to themselves, and the distinction between true and false progressively loses its contours, and man ends by fully believing the story he has told so many times and continues to tell, polishing and retouching here and there the details which are least credible or incongruous or incompatible with the acquired picture of historically accepted events; initial bad faith has become good faith. The silent transition from falsehood to self-deception is useful: anyone who lies in good faith is better off. He recites his part better, is more easily believed by the judge, the historian, the reader, his wife, and his children. (pp. 26–27)

Levi noted that people can fabricate a convenient reality, which is told and retold to oneself, until the fact that it was once a fabrication is authentically forgotten. It then can be presented to the world as truth with felt sincerity. Levi addressed this squarely as a moral choice for which a person is fully responsible, not excused by any role unconscious processes play in its genesis or sustenance.

In a different vein, Robert Jay Lifton (1986) in *The Nazi Doctors* described
"doubling" as a psychological coping mechanism that enabled Nazi physicians
to participate in torture, murder, and genocide in German death camps. He
noted evidence that these doctors were not psychiatrically ill. They also had
not been violent or brutal men in their personal histories or at home in their
families and communities. Rather, they wrapped their deeds in Nazi ideology,
explaining that as physicians they were curing their Nordic race of disease by
terminating, sometimes in grotesque medical experiments, the lives of Jewish,
Roma (Gypsy), mentally ill, developmentally disabled, homosexual, and other
"defectives." Doubling was a coping mechanism that permitted a Nazi doctor
to embrace fully the demands of his ideological group while preserving a sense
of self as an ethical, conscientious, responsible professional. As a Nazi doctor,
Fritz Klein justified his role: "Of course I am a doctor and I want to preserve
life. And out of respect for human life, I would remove a gangrenous appendix from a diseased body. The Jew is the gangrenous appendix in the body of
mankind" (Lifton, 1986, p. 16).

Lifton (1986) described doubling as a psychological mechanism through
which the self dissociatively splits into "two functioning wholes, so that a
part-self acts as an entire self" (p. 418). He listed five features of doubling that
might also detail progression, in Levi's terms, to the bad faith of self-deception
(p. 419):

1. Doubling exists as a dialectic between the two selves in terms of
   autonomy and connection. A Nazi doctor "needed his Auschwitz self
   to function psychologically in an environment so antithetical to his
   previous ethic standards. At the same time, he needed his prior self in
   order to continue seeing himself as human physician, husband, father.
   The Auschwitz self had to be both autonomous and connected to the
   prior self."
2. Doubling follows a holistic principle. That is, the Auschwitz self could
   fully embrace the perceptions, emotions, values, and actions of the
   Auschwitz death camp.
3. Doubling has a life–death dimension, experienced as a survival strategy. That is, a "killing self" emerged protectively, acting on behalf of
   one's healing or survival.
4. Doubling avoids the felt experience of guilt. Only the second self does
   evil deeds, which subsequently are not owned by the prior self as its
   own experience.
5. Doubling involves unconscious processes. These mechanisms largely
   operate outside awareness of choice and moral decision making.

"Unspeakable dilemmas" have been associated with medically unexplained symptoms, such as headaches, vomiting, seizures, weakness, or numbness that have no discoverable medical cause (Griffith & Griffith, 1994; Griffith, Polles, & Griffith, 1998). An unspeakable dilemma is a situation in which a person feels intolerably trapped between desires and obligations, or between expectations of self and expectations of others, but where the kind of dialogue necessary for resolving the dilemma is prohibited. Unbearable distress whose expression feels forbidden is a common social context in which somatization occurs. Shame, humiliation, guilt, and threats of harm to self or others are frequent reasons why discussions of unspeakable dilemmas are prohibited for those involved. A somatized symptom can be regarded as the body's silent protest, a public performance of an unspeakable dilemma (Griffith & Griffith, 1994).

Bad faith, doubling, and unspeakable dilemmas survey similar territory from different angles. They share similarities but show differences in focus. Bad faith and doubling describe how normal dissociative processes can support externalized violence against outgroups. Unspeakable dilemmas describe how normal dissociative processes can support an internalized silencing of self that generates "as if" symptoms of physical illness.

Bad faith illuminates the role of human volition, an active choice for self-deception, to comply with, rather than to rebel against, social forces coercing immoral acts. It is about ethics. Doubling, as a social psychology construct, presents an economic model of a whole person who uses both conscious and unconscious self-deception to accommodate an immoral world while conserving some sense of oneself as a moral person. An unspeakable dilemma is a first-person statement of existential experience, spoken by a person's suppressed self: "I am trapped without a voice other than my physical symptoms of illness."

Bad faith, doubling, and unspeakable dilemmas each articulate how hardwired dissociative capabilities of human brains can be used in intended and unintended ways to sustain sociobiological connections to one's social world, while conserving some remnant of selfhood. As solutions, they each work imperfectly and sometimes at high costs.

Normal dissociative processes have long been employed by religious and ideological groups in order to render group members pliable to directives flowing from group identity, group hierarchy and roles, and processes of social exchange, sometimes sacrificing the needs of individuals. As Karen Armstrong (2004) noted about her training as a novitiate:

> The training was designed to make us wholly self-reliant, so that we no longer needed human love or approval. We too were told that we were to

die to our old selves and to our worldly, secular way of looking at things. Of course, we were not buried alive in a tomb or anything of that sort, but we were constantly undermined, belittled, publicly castigated, or ordered to do things that were patently absurd. As Ignatius's Rule put it, we were to become utterly pliable to the will of God, as expressed through our superiors, in the same way as "a dead body allows itself to be treated in any manner whatever, or as an old man's stick serves him who holds it in every place and for every use alike." Dead to ourselves, we would live a fuller, enhanced existence. (pp. 27–28)

Practical Limits of Dissociative Self-Silencing as a Coping Style

Suppressing personal self through dissociative processes comes with substantial costs for individuals. Dissociative suppression of emotional responses does not necessarily spare the body from physiological stress (Benham & Younger, 2008, pp. 421–422). Further, prolonged suppression of emotional reactivity usually produces emotional numbing like that of depersonalization disorder, not pleasure or contentment (Simeon & Abugel, 2006). Repeated choices to suppress personal feelings often end in numbness even when a person is fully aware of good reasons for the choices. Those who have resigned themselves to feigned acceptance of roles or relationships that, in fact, feel like self-betrayal often report, "I stopped feeling anything." Like morning mist under the sun, a capacity to feel life richly and fully vanishes as acts of emotional suppression become routinized and habitual.

People in circumstances that demand conformity to group or organizational standards thus can appear dull, empty, and emotionally distanced from themselves and other people. In their docility, however, such individuals can enact group agendas, including abusive, exploitive, neglectful, or sadistic ones, that they could never enact as moral, reflective individuals away from the group.

Exploiting the Instability of Dissociative Self-Silencing in Clinical Interventions

Dissociative processes associated with bad faith, doubling, and unspeakable dilemmas usually are only partially effective in sequestering self-awareness of a personal self. Focused attention and suppression of emotional responses must be sustained to maintain dissociation. Validity of shaming and humiliating judgments must stay unquestioned. From one hour to the next, dissociative processes fluctuate in the extent to which they can keep information belonging to each of the two selves compartmentalized. The hidden observer always stands in the background of awareness as a threat to robot-like obedience. Dissociative silencing of a personal self and its emotional responsiveness is typically partial and unstable. Its effects are not fixed or permanent.

Cohesive religious and ideological groups constantly must work to keep energized a sense of group identity and rigid boundaries necessary to keep the outside world at a distance. They intensify dominance/submission, peer affiliation, and reciprocal altruism processes, while expressing a dismissive attitude toward personal selves. This steadfast expenditure of individual and group energies is difficult to sustain over long periods of time. Lapses in dissociative suppression and fatigue from the ongoing mental work required to sustain them can create openings for undermining their operations. Subsequent chapters illustrate how such openings can provide beachheads from which dialogues can be initiated that can help liberate a personal self and rediscover lost capacities for personal spirituality.

7

✦

Asserting Primacy
of Personal Spirituality
over Sociobiological Religion

AN INDIVIDUAL PERSON MATTERS MORE THAN HIS OR HER *yes + no*
social identity, role, status, or functional use in society; this is the central
message of personal spirituality. Whole-person relatedness is fundamentally
incompatible with bad faith or doubling. Emotional postures of resilience—
coherency, hope, communion, purpose, commitment—undermine the power
of social constraints that produce unspeakable dilemmas.

When personal spirituality strengthens, the religious world of sociobiology does not disappear. However, it is domesticated to serve the well-being of ✓
individual persons. The role of sociobiological religion is transformed. Personal spirituality tends to recruit secure attachment styles rather than anxious *yes*
or avoidant ones. Social hierarchy and peer affiliation processes are refocused
to attend first to needs of individual members of religious groups rather than
group missions. Ms. Johnson, in the Introduction, exemplified a person with
a strong personal spirituality who also participated actively in her church
community with its hierarchy, roles, and social expectations. This was not
so for Ms. Ames, whose illness was driven by her faithful submissiveness in
her church and its doctrinal teachings. Her recovery from illness began with
a rekindling of personal spirituality that eventually made her relationship *NB*
with God primary and obedience to ecclesiastical authority secondary. As a

141

therapeutic strategy, strengthening personal spirituality counters most religious processes that do harm when their sociobiological behaviors are taken to excess. Designing clinical interventions to achieve this aim relies upon an accurate appraisal of sociobiological and neurobiological factors evident in the initial clinical encounter.

Tailoring Interventions Informed by Sociobiology and Neurobiology

When clinical concerns have been raised about a patient's religious life, a clinician greeting the patient may meet a defensive wall of sociobiological behaviors that block person-to-person contact: dismissiveness, belittlement, monologues referencing scriptures or ideological talking points, refusals by religious group members to leave the patient alone with the clinician. Sociobiological and neurobiological perspectives do not replace well-composed psychodynamic, cognitive-behavioral, or family systems formulations of clinical problems, but rather add to them. Sociobiological and neurobiological perspectives can help guide the staging of clinical encounters so that they start successfully.

Sociobiological and neurobiological perspectives can provide empathic guidance for organizing interactions that favor collaboration and dialogue. They can help a clinician to anticipate what is reasonable or unreasonable to expect from a patient or family in terms of change. They can help a clinician to be aware of pitfalls during interactions and to avoid precipitous breakdowns. Sometimes clinical interventions must be conducted under a limited and conditional therapeutic alliance. At times they must be conducted under a truce, but no therapeutic alliance. Sometimes clinician and patient must work together as "strange bedfellows" (Herzig & Chasin, 2006) because there are no good alternatives, as when a patient otherwise religiously disdainful of psychiatry must rely on a psychiatric consultant's advocacy in order to refuse unwanted medical treatment on religious grounds. Sociobiological and neurobiological perspectives can help provide a more nuanced understanding of religious behavior as is required for clinical work conducted with ambivalent and tenuous treatment relationships.

For dialogue to be viable, preliminary capacity-building interventions may need to occur at two levels simultaneously: First, to open space externally for expression of personal spirituality by tempering the influence of sociobiological elements that would suppress it; second, to support the influence of personal spirituality interiorly within the patient's conscious awareness. For this work, a clinician must find a therapeutic position close enough to learn about the patient's experiential world but not so close as to raise alarm.

Dual Interventions: Challenging Both Externalizing Sociobiological and Internalizing Dissociative Processes

Dual interventions may be necessary to target both overreaching sociobiological systems (interpersonally) and dissociative suppression (intrapersonally). How much interpersonal and how much intrapersonal varies case to case. Some self-aware individuals easily recollect past experiences when a marriage, church, or society placed emotional strictures that impoverished their lives. When helped to see with clarity the dimensions of a current unspeakable dilemma, they move assertively to change their circumstances without further assistance from a clinician. Other individuals have lived so long in existences programmed by roles, loyalties, and obligations that locating a hidden-away sense of self and combating dissociative numbing become the major focus of clinical work.

The Loneliest Profession: A Pastor's Wife

Ms. Simpson was a 27-year-old pastor's wife who was hospitalized for sudden paralysis, which had raised fears that she had a stroke. When neurological studies were normal, her neurologist sought psychiatric consultation to determine whether her weakness had emotional origins. Ms. Simpson carried too many job descriptions. She was mother of three children ages 5, 3, and 1 year and, as the pastor's wife, also worked in a supportive role at the church. Since their church was too small to support a full-time pastor's salary, both she and her husband worked other full-time jobs. This, of course, meant that she had a 5-day (Monday–Friday) workweek juxtaposed against a weekend routine of church work that peaked with the Sunday morning church services.

Ms. Simpson's husband had entered the ministry only a year earlier. As a young minister, his ideas differed from those of the older church members. There were also competitive factions within the small membership of the church. Ms. Simpson tried to listen to her husband's struggles and to support him.

"Your husband has a wife to listen to him. Who listens to you?" I asked. She smiled and said quietly, "No one." She missed her parents and friends in her old community. Parishioners could not substitute as confidants.

Despite their overloaded schedules, Ms. Simpson and her husband had a mutual agreement that "church stays at church"; they wouldn't bring church problems home to their personal space. However, one Sunday, her mother-in-law called with advice for her son on how to manage his church problems. The young pastor was furious with his mother, and Ms. Simpson resented her mother-in-law's meddling, feeling that church frustrations were now intruding into her home. This marked the day when her physical symptoms started occurring.

As I summarized my hearing of her story, Ms. Simpson listened thoughtfully. Shaking her head, she acknowledged how angry she felt. I noted how difficult it was to deal not only with multiple sets of demands but also with the political constraints, which meant she had to edit what could be said within which church and family relationships. There was no one with whom she could spontaneously and freely express herself. This was her unspeakable dilemma: Not only did she feel trapped in an intolerable position, but she did not feel free to disclose the existence of her problem. She chose silence instead.

Ms. Simpson and her husband agreed to meet as a couple with a counselor to address these issues together. Their aim would be to draw a clear boundary about their marriage and home, separating it from intrusions by church problems. Ms. Simpson's strong sense of self and comfortable assertiveness made it easy to imagine that she could successfully establish boundaries and set needed limits once she felt convinced that this would be best for all involved.

God's Wounded Warrior

Mr. Burns, a thin, young man, sat up vigilantly in his bed, scrutinizing me as I entered his room. I explained that his neurologist had been unable to find a cause for the episodes of tremors and incoordination that led to his hospitalization. His neurologist wondered whether stress in his life might be contributing to his symptoms and wanted me to help reveal the answer to that question. Mr. Burns reluctantly consented to the interview.

I reviewed Mr. Burns's medical story as it had been delineated in his hospital chart. He had struggled with severe diabetes since childhood. In his 20s, he had a rash of physical injuries as well as gastrointestinal and urinary tract symptoms for which definitive diagnoses could not be established despite lengthy medical evaluations. The medical evaluations had failed to find diagnoses for some of his recent symptoms: nausea, chest pain, irregular heartbeats. I asked what his best sense was regarding the cause of these symptoms. He angrily told me how his internist had confronted him with an abrupt accusation that "there is nothing wrong with you," after medical tests reported normal findings. Mr. Burns felt stunned, betrayed, and bitterly angry. He dismissed the doctor from his case, but then felt lost and confused as to where to turn next.

He then told about his current symptoms. He was having shaking tremors that seemed to be triggered by pressure against his spine. He feared that this was the consequence of an old sports injury. I commented that he was shouldering a large burden: Diabetes was a chronic disease that required more and more care as one aged, and it must take a lot of work to manage this plus the disconcerting episodes of jerking, especially since the doctor to whom he had turned had been of no help. What kept him from giving up or being overwhelmed? "My faith in God," Mr. Burns responded.

"Do you feel the presence of God as you go through this?" I asked, wanting to know whether he meant faith as an abstract belief in God or as a felt emotional presence of God.

"No," he responded. "My faith is in God."

Unsure whether he understood my question, I reworded it. "I mean, can you tell the difference between moments when God feels close or when He feels far away? Can you tell the difference?"

"I don't feel God's presence. I have faith in God."

This stood out to me as a distinction of importance, because it seemed to omit a sense of his emotional relatedness with God. I asked a third question to try to clarify. "If you talk with a range of Christians, I think you will find some people who say 'My faith is a belief, a confidence in God,' but others will say 'I know God is with me because I feel God to be with me.'"

"That is immature faith," he responded. "Feelings are of the flesh." With a dismissive tone, he added, "I pay no attention to feelings one way or the other."

I heard this as a reflection of his attitude about feelings generally, an attitude that I anticipated would extend beyond his relationship with God. I responded, "Physicians worry about how emotional stress can hinder the functioning of the brain. That is why they are often concerned about a person's feelings."

"If you have diabetes, you learn not to pay attention to what you feel," Mr. Burns answered. "You may be feeling depressed, but you check your glucose and it's low; you take in sugar, you feel better. You feel it is a great day, but your glucose is high and that is why. You can't trust feelings."

I pressed him. "The flesh is with you," I said. "As long as you are living, you live in relationship with your material body. What is the short list for the areas in which you most struggle with the flesh?"

He then quoted a verse of scripture in which a long list of vices of the flesh were named. Lust, anger, and envy were the three that he most struggled with.

I then stated a hypothesis, carefully presenting it in a subjunctive "what if" sense and within a religious metaphor: Perhaps he was locked in spiritual warfare between his desire to live a life of the spirit and the desires of the flesh. The tension produced might be making his body ill. He seemed to follow the logic of this but again responded with another quotation from the Bible, a scripture verse from St. Paul calling upon Christians to beat the flesh into submission.

I sensed that Mr. Burns experienced me to be respectful of his personal dignity and religious faith. Buttressed by this, I felt I could venture further in challenging him. "The problem as I see it is that beating into submission may not be a good way to relate to something that you can't get out of your life."

"Are you telling me you think I should let the flesh take over?" he asked curtly.

"No. I'm just suggesting there might be other possibilities beside beating the flesh into submission or letting the flesh take over. Like riding a horse—a good rider rides with the horse. He doesn't try to force the horse, nor does he let the horse go where the horse wants to go. I am concerned that as you have tried to exert tighter and tighter control over your feelings, the struggle and tension have increased, not lessened, and they are making your body ill."

"What are you suggesting then?" Mr. Burns asked.

"If this idea has any merit, then I would recommend that you work with someone who can understand what you are struggling with, not try to do it alone. Psychotherapy with a mental health professional who understands and respects your faith could be one option. Perhaps seeing a pastoral counselor who understands how a spiritual struggle might make the body ill could be another possibility. I'll bet you know Christians who do not have this kind of warfare going on within them. If you were to spend time with someone who is older and has lived a lot of years, there might be things you could learn."

I left him with my card and told him I would be glad to meet with him in the future if he chose. We shook hands and parted on what felt to be a friendly note.

My bedside interview was narrowly focused upon the patient's individual participation in the process of illness. Clinically, Mr. Burns's physical symptoms would be regarded as somatic dissociation, commonly termed a "conversion disorder." I felt there was good evidence that he customarily utilized dissociative suppression of his normal emotional responsiveness to cope with distressful feelings, but that this was now failing him. His symptoms could be understood metaphorically as his body's protest, a rebellion against a totalitarian control he tried to exert over it. However, I was aware that there was another unaddressed context adding to my difficulties in responding fully.

The social context of his symptoms was largely a religious one. He was a member of a Protestant fundamentalist "Bible church." I assumed that the theology of his church reinforced his efforts to suppress negative emotions through strong beliefs. I knew that he was being counseled by a pastor who advocated this approach to managing his life. Both church and pastor would likely steer him away from mental health professionals like myself, whose work would be suspect, which is why I suggested he "spend time with someone older and has lived a lot of years." A psychologically mature elder in his church might be better positioned for this role than a mental health professional. He likely would feel discredited and shamed if his peers in the church were to learn that he was meeting with a psychiatrist because that would be evidence that he was unable to manage his emotional conflicts as a Christian man.

Could I have gone further therapeutically? It was my assessment that his relationship to church leaders, his peer relations within his Christian community, and his ethical sense of Biblical living all supported, rather than challenged, his silencing of his feelings and spontaneity. When the vicissitudes of friendships, a romantic relationship, and his professional ambitions had produced anxieties and uncertainties, he met them with "the rule," as Karen Armstrong (see Chapter 6) was taught in the convent: to discredit and to disregard his spontaneous thoughts and impulses, attending only to the marching orders he perceived as godly.

It was my judgment that in this interview I could not ask questions about the religious community in which Mr. Burns lived. He had uneasily opened the interior of his life to me. I felt much like a stranger permitted to enter a family home out of courtesy but still watched closely and warily. Was I friend or foe? In small moves, I had steadily pushed the limits of what could be questioned. I closely attended to not just his words but to his tensed muscles, his breathing, and his gaze to tell me how far I could venture in this initial interview. I felt reasonably sure that any efforts to call into question the recommendations from his peers, pastor, and religious doctrines would have simply stopped the conversation. This was where future conversations with others might need to go.

Moral Reasoning in Religious Life

Rebalancing the relative influences of religious sociobiology and personal spirituality brings clinical treatment into a moral discourse. Helping a person to value one's personal experience is not simply a step toward mental health or emotional maturity but also an ethical choice. Choosing to prioritize one's individual feelings does not happen in a social vacuum. It impacts relationships with other people, sometimes with painful consequences for others affected. It changes one's identity as a person. Mr. Burns's intuitive wariness might well have been on target, in that the structure of his relational and assumptive world might have been at risk had he chosen to enter with me whole-heartedly into a more open exploration of his emotional responses.

Helping an individual reassert a personal self against the prescriptions and prohibitions of society has long been a mission of Western psychotherapy. Reduced to simplest elements, most psychotherapy consists of four steps: helping a person (1) to notice his or her emotional experiences, (2) to find language for them, (3) to have conversations about them, and (4) to make experientially informed changes in perceptions, thoughts, and behaviors that lead to a more gratifying life. What has been too often missing from psychotherapy, however, has been the moral context for this decision making.

Suffering can be due not only to psychopathology—disordered brains, psychodynamic conflicts, or dysfunctional family systems that make suffering obligatory—but also to actions in accord with deeply held values or commitments. Sometimes a self-aware person, such as Mother Theresa or Thomas Merton, chooses a path of self-renunciation out of commitment to God or compassion toward others. An Ayn Rand-like individualism is not necessarily the best outcome for "what is the right thing to do." Expectations drawn from social hierarchy, kin recognition, peer affiliation, and fair social exchange are also important sources that people rely on when deciding what is the right thing to do. This rebalancing of personal spirituality and sociobiological religion must be carefully deliberated, honoring a patient's commitments and giving sociobiology its due while also asking questions from a world outside those commitments and sociobiology.

Mr. Chin: No Option for a Clinician to Intervene

In the Introduction, Mr. Chin presented a clinical dilemma around refusal of needed orthopedic surgery because of his religious faith. He faced the possibility of a lifelong physical disability if he refused the surgery, but his primary concern was a moral one: What was the right thing to do? He turned for guidance to his Fulan Gong beliefs and the peer affiliation of his community. The solidarity he felt within his religious community supplanted concern for his individual well-being. I had no vantage point from which to inquire about personal spirituality that might diverge from the expectations and prescribed behaviors of his religious group. I also had no collaborative relationship with the Fulan Gong community through which I might have worked in a both/and manner, which might have enabled respect for Mr. Chin's religious identity while still permitting him to receive biomedical treatment. In the end, I acted in accordance with my understanding of the law and medical ethics, which directed me to respect his right to make choices even if they were in opposition to the medical recommendations and what I would have wished for him.

Chilean biologist Humberto Maturana (Maturana & Varela, 1992) used an evolutionary perspective to propose that the fundamental meaning of love within the animal kingdom is simply to make space for the other, to let the other live alongside, to permit the other to live as an autonomous creature. There are situations where a clinician lacks the knowledge, skills, creativity, or opportunity to do more than that in attempts to heal or to relieve suffering. When few openings can be created for human relatedness in greater depth, simply making space for the other remains as a basement-level clinical imperative.

Ms. Bridges: Consultant to Her Sociobiological Religious Life

Mr. Chin can be contrasted with Ms. Bridges, a member of the Jehovah's Witnesses faith who also was refusing medical recommendations. Ms. Bridges had been admitted to our hospital for severe, uncontrolled hypertension that placed her at risk for stroke or heart attack. She was refusing to take medication to control her blood pressure. Her internist asked for a psychiatric consultation to determine whether she had the decision-making capacity to refuse. There were fears that she might be delusional and psychotic, so intense and irrational seemed her religious ideology and her disregard of her health. There was a growing consensus among her clinicians that medical treatment should be forced involuntarily, if that were the only way for her hypertension to be treated.

When I met Ms. Bridges, I doubted the diagnosis of psychosis but realized how one might have concluded that. Before even learning my name, she was expounding, in fast sentences and using no commas, the tenets of her religious faith. Hearing this as a ritualistic greeting, a "cultural handshake" within her religious group, I listened quietly, then sat down beside her and asked if we could talk. She told me about her belief in the sovereignty of God and her love for Jesus. I explained that the medical team was worried both about the seriousness of her hypertension and that the treatment might not fit with her beliefs. She responded graciously, seeming glad that I wanted to sit and talk. As we discussed the disagreement over her medication, she clarified that her concern was about receiving blood products. The word "blood" in "high blood pressure medicine" disturbed her. I asked if she would consider taking it if there were a guarantee that it would contain no blood products. She said this might be possible. Her response pointed to a region of ambiguity where there might be room for negotiation.

I wondered how much she personally knew about hypertension. She said that she and her siblings had been left in the care of a foster mother until she was 12 years old. Her foster mother was obese and hypertensive. This recollection of her foster mother brought forth a sudden flood of bad memories and stories about her foster mother's rages and neglect of the children ("She was a mix between Joan Crawford and Bette Davis"). When the conversation eventually returned to her hypertension, I learned that she had never known any one with kidney disease, heart disease, stroke, or other serious complications of untreated hypertension. Hypertension thus lacked any fear factor in motivating her concern about it. "I talk with God, and he calms me," was her preferred strategy for dealing with her hypertension, a commonly held but naïve view that emotional upset creates high blood pressure, as she believed happened with her foster mother.

I asked how conflicts between medical care and her church's teachings could be negotiated. She described how the church could issue document papers stating its position on her medical care. So long as there was no transfer of blood products, she did not think the church elders would pose objections. "Jesus is watching, minding what I'm saying," she said. "You can make me survive up to a point, but Jesus watches over me. Jesus knows what I'm thinking when I sleep, he knows what I'm thinking when I get up. I pray and try to be obedient."

I listened to the tone of security in her attachment to Jesus and moved to align myself both with it and with her church roles and affiliations that gave her life stability. I said we were concerned about how we could help her survive up to that point where her faith took over. Did she feel that our medical care was in accordance with God's leadership? She said she had been treated well at our hospital and felt the doctors were "walking along with God." I wondered how she discerned that. "When a person is gentle, kind, calm, not quick to anger, I know they walk with God" she said. I clarified, "That is how you know you might know whether I, as a doctor, might also walk with God?" "Yes," she responded.

At this point, it appeared possible that taking antihypertensive medication could occur within the scope of her religious faith. I asked whether she had a primary care physician to oversee her care. She said that her previous doctor had retired. She lived in senior housing and was unsure how to locate a new primary care physician. This led to a plan. First, her medical team would provide her with a written statement that her antihypertensive medications did not involve any exchange of blood products. Second, we would communicate to her church elders that their help was needed in organizing her outpatient medical care and ensuring that she attended visits to her new primary care doctor.

My encounter with Ms. Bridges did not attempt to change the structure of her religious world or her relationship to it. Space for dialogue and negotiation opened when she felt respect for her religious identity and my interest in learning more about it. Structuring an interaction simply to favor dialogue is not an instrumental intervention, yet it can be a potent one. My presence, listening, helping her search for a solution that would enable acceptance of medical treatment, while leaving her religious beliefs untouched, made a difference that she acknowledged. My status as a psychiatrist was still that of a noncitizen within her realm. I was a foreign power with benevolent intentions. We could partner, agreeing to disagree about our worldviews and still accomplish the task of her health. As she said, this was how she decided whether a person walked with God.

Ms. Ames: Reasserting Personal Spirituality within a World of Sociobiological Religion

Ms. Ames, in the Introduction, was someone for whom clinical options opened more fully than for either Mr. Chin or Ms. Bridges. What was possible therapeutically extended beyond simply expressing respect or partnering across differences. Ms. Ames opened her religious world and granted me permission to inquire about its constitution. Rather than a single-session consultation, we could work in a steady-paced manner in regular psychotherapy. The work of the therapy was dually focused, both upon loosening the hold of sociobiological religion over her personal self and on stoking the coals of a reemergent person-centered spirituality.

Ms. Ames's clinical problem, nonepileptic seizures and other psychosomatic symptoms, had been associated with religious submission that progressively had stifled her sense of a personal self. Elsewhere in her life, she was assertive and had competed to achieve success in a demanding career. In marriage and religious life, however, her commitment was an unquestioning obedience that flowed from a traditionally Catholic interpretation of roles, rules, and responsibilities as a wife. Her husband heaped ridicule upon her whenever she fell short of his expectations. She did not challenge the power asymmetry in their relationship. As her husband became more coercive in his abuse, she devoted even greater energy toward duty, obedience, and self-silencing until the point where she became psychosomatically ill.

Her turn toward health came when she sensed God's validation that care of self took priority over the church's specifications for marriage. This occurred in an epiphany that she interpreted as a direct communication from God. When her neurologist diagnosed her seizures as stress induced, she experienced this as a jarring "wake-up call from God."

Ms. Ames's psychotherapy covered a larger expanse than only her religious life. The latter was central, however. Over the course of 20 sessions, she articulated four tenets felt to be consistent with her spirituality but divergent from her former equating of godliness with obedience and submission:

+ "My illness is a wake-up call from God."
+ "I believe I should live my life in the way God meant it to be lived. God meant us to be happy people."
+ "God wants me to care for my health, to take care of my body."
+ "If I don't take responsibility for taking care of my health, it will be taken away."

Her husband initially responded to her new care of self by escalating his anger and demands. She made a firm and definitive end to the marriage. She embraced exercise, hobbies, travel, and relationships in a new program for care of self. She did not leave her Christian faith, though, nor did she change any specific religious beliefs. Rather, figure and ground reversed between personal spirituality and the sociobiological dimensions of her religious life, with the former moving center stage. As she later commented, "I'm not 100% Catholic—there are God-made laws and man-made laws. I don't agree with all the man-made laws of the Catholic Church."

Near the end of her psychotherapy, I asked, "What would you say that you have learned about your life over the past couple of years?"

"I would say that I learned that I have to take care of myself," she responded.

"But what does that mean? What do you notice differently or think about?" I asked.

"There are small hurts and large hurts," she answered.

"And when there are large hurts, you take note of that in a way you did not a year ago?" I followed.

"You can feel it in your body that you are getting sick," she said.

"What do you do?" I asked.

"Well, my faith—I pray every day for God to guide the way," she responded.

"How do you discern God's guidance? Do you hear God's voice or see a sign?" I asked.

"No, I feel it inside me," she answered.

"Where?" I wondered.

"Here, inside me," she responded, moving her hand over her lower chest and abdomen.

"So you don't hear God's voice or see something that tells you. You listen to God within your body?" I asked.

"You feel it when you are getting sick," she said.

"Little hurts you can live with. Big hurts make you sick?" I restated.

"Yes," she answered.

Ms. Ames worked out the full implications of this transformation over a 2-year span of psychotherapy. However, the epiphany that set these changes in motion—experiencing her symptoms as a "wake-up call from God"—seemed to happen in a moment. The context for change perhaps had been already set by her neurologist. No doubt her hidden observer for some time had been taking stock inwardly. Her neurologist identified her husband's berating as not only abusive but also causative of symptoms. When her neurologist stepped forward as her ally, the isolation required to maintain dissociative silencing of self was ruptured. Her religious sociobiology was checked in its advances. She began choosing right and wrong in a different way.

Intrapersonal Politics of Religious Life

Sociobiological systems create a relational meshwork through which family religiousness and societal religious groups can reach deeply into the heart of an individual person. The critical question is whether this reach produces a protective shade under which personal spirituality flourishes or whether the shade stunts its growth because of lack of light. Religious organizations and their leaders sometimes use the sociobiological domains of religion irresponsibly to manage the emotional hearts of individuals without concern for their individual lives. Sometimes well-meaning religious groups and families stifle personal spirituality in their zeal to teach and to protect. A religiously over-managed life is vulnerable to a host of psychiatric and psychosomatic ills, as the vignettes of these chapters attest.

What is the end game? Should a clinician make it a mission to help patients dismember their sociobiological religiousness, replacing it with a robust personal spirituality? The picture that is brought to mind is of a wandering monk, ascetic, begging alms, praying constantly, extending compassion to others, and caring not a whit for the social roles, hierarchies, or group loyalties that largely characterize the world's religions and its societies. Is there good that can come from the sociobiology of religion?

My personal image of a good outcome came from a clinical encounter with Ms. Jasper, whom I met at her hospital bedside after she had been struck by a hit-and-run driver while she was crossing the street at a crosswalk. For 5 years, she had struggled with physical disabilities from multiple sclerosis. The driver evidently did not see her moving slowly across the street, hit her, and fled in panic. Bystanders rescued her and called 911. Still recovering in the hospital 4 weeks later, her rehabilitation doctor worried about the impact of the accident on her emotional well-being and asked me to see her.

Ms. Jasper greeted me courteously. I explained why I had come and that I was aware of both her multiple sclerosis and recent physical injuries.

"It sounds like the past 4 weeks with surgery for your broken leg have been hard," I commented.

"Yes, it has been terrible," she said.

I asked whether she had ever been through anything like this before. "Never," she responded.

"At this point in time, what is your greatest concern?"

"Becoming mobile," she said. "If I'm not able to drive, I won't be able to keep my job." She was remembering how long it had taken for her right leg to recover during previous physical rehabilitation for an exacerbation of her multiple sclerosis. It had been usable but weak and stiff ever since. She was afraid that the addition of a fracture meant she would not be able to drive a car.

"How does the fear present itself?" I asked. She told how she had merely read the words "wheelchair bound" and heard the words "nursing home." Now these phrases were returning involuntarily as traumatic, intrusive images that evoked her fear.

"How much is fear and how much is discouragement?" I asked, wanting to draw a finer distinction between posttraumatic fear and a demoralized mood.

"I'm not discouraged," she responded. "I pray constantly."

"Can you tell me the words of your prayer?" I asked.

"The Lord is my Shepherd, I shall not want . . . the 23rd psalm. And sometimes I recite the 68th psalm." She repeated a portion of an additional prayer she had memorized. Her body fell still and her emotions quietened as she spoke. Recitation of these scriptures and prayers evidently were her spiritual practices.

"Do you also say prayers to God that are requests?" I asked.

"Yes, I pray for healing," she responded.

"Do you sense that God hears your prayers?" I wondered.

"Yes," she said.

"Do you feel God's presence? I mean, you have faith in God, and you believe God hears your prayer. Do you actually feel God's presence?" I asked.

"Yes," she responded, "I pray constantly."

"Are there some times when you don't feel God's presence?" I asked.

She laughed. "Yes. I teach junior high students. When I'm in the middle of it at school, God feels far away."

"And when God feels close . . . How do you sense that inside yourself?" I asked.

"I just feel happy inside. I feel like hope is alive," she responded.

"How else do you manage fear?" I asked, returning to the symptom that was resisting her management.

"Many in my church are also praying. And my family visits—my two daughters," she answered. I realized that as much as my questions were focused upon her personal and intimate experiences of spirituality, she likely relied as much upon the doctrinal traditions of her Christian faith and the communal support of her church and family.

"This may be a question that is too soon to ask, but is there anything that going through this experience has added to your life?" I queried.

She told how she had been in a confused state after the accident from her head injury. She had little memory of it. However, her daughter told her that she slipped in and out of prayer, even though confused where she was at the time. "I have a testimony," she said.

I asked what she wanted people to hear in her testimony. "That prayer keeps hope alive," she responded. She told how she could tell the story to her students, and they would be able to see that faith can carry a person through hard times.

Who would not resent the hit-and-run driver? Who might not hate God for failing to protect, first against multiple sclerosis but certainly against the randomness of careless drivers? Who would not feel bitterly the absence of a just world in which good people are struck down and bad ones flee crime scenes with no punishment? I cannot say Ms. Jasper did not pass through each of these emotional responses at some point. When she and I met, however, it seemed clear that she had staked her own position toward the universe and now stood by it. She had made the turn from resentment to gratitude.

There is no evidence that religious faith will spare a person from posttraumatic symptoms after being run down by a car. There is evidence suggesting that recovery is speeded and risk of chronicity lessened when a robust personal spirituality is also supported by traditional religious practices, doctrinal beliefs, and a caring community that make up the sociobiological dimensions of formal religion. Ms. Jasper's posttraumatic intrusive images might have warranted additional specific treatment, but she did not leave the hospital as a traumatized person. In the best way, Ms. Jasper presented her personal spirituality and sociobiological religious life as working in harmony, each serving a role in furthering her recovery.

My role as a clinician was small in size but possibly important for Ms. Jasper. One could imagine many different narratives that could have been constructed from the bare facts of Ms. Jasper's anxiety symptoms and medical history. With my questions and listening, I helped her articulate the story that she most wanted to tell. A narrative coherently composed, spoken, and witnessed by others is more likely to be recollected and incorporated into one's identity (White, 2007; Weingarten, 2003). As a mental health professional, I stood as a particular kind of witness. For better or worse, acknowledgment by a medical professional is often experienced by patients as a particular warranting of a story's importance (Slavney, 1999). From her suffering, Ms. Jasper received a narrative of faith and prayer—a testimony—that would be shared with family, friends, and, above all, her junior high students.

A secular clinician can play an important role by helping a patient to push back the reach of sociobiological religion in order to open space for personal spirituality that can replenish whole persons, both the patient and other people. When personal spirituality is vibrant, then the sociobiological domains of religion can resettle into useful roles that continue to protect and support people as unique individuals.

8

The Religious Who Protect
Only Their Own
Clinical Problems from Peer Affiliation,
Kin Recognition, and Social Exchange

IMMACULEE ILIBAGIZA WAS A YOUNG RWANDAN TUTSI STUDENT
in 1994 when she and seven other Tutsi women survived 91 days hidden in a
closet-sized bathroom of a Hutu Protestant pastor's home during the Rwanda
genocide (Ilibagiza, 2006). Machete-wielding Hutu gangs, which included
former friends and schoolmates, looked for them, twice searching the home
where they were hidden. More than 800,000 Tutsis throughout the country,
including Immaculee's other family members, were slaughtered. Emaciated but
alive, she survived against all odds under Pastor Murinzi's protection. Yet the
story was far more complex than this bare story line.

The context for ethnic conflict in Rwanda had been set by the Belgian
colonial government, who considered the taller height and the facial features of the Tutsis to be more physically attractive by European standards and
favored them for positions within the educational and governmental institutions. After Rwanda gained independence, resentments of the majority Hutu
population spilled over into indiscriminate violence against the Tutsis in
1959 and 1973, causing hundreds of thousands of Tutsis to flee the country. In
1994, expatriot Tutsi rebels were organizing the Rwandese Patriotic Front and
threatening to invade and retake the country from the Hutus. In response,

Hutu extremists planned a preemptive surprise attack on Tutsis still living within the country that would quickly erase their 14% of the population.

Pastor Murinzi faced a moral dilemma on the night when Immaculee fled to his home pleading for protection. He was Hutu. Further, he identified with the grievances and shared the fears of his Hutu kinsmen. Immaculee was Catholic and he was Protestant; she was not a member of a particular church congregation for which he was responsible. He also held certain personal resentments against Immaculee's father, who had been a community leader. Most of all, he had a wife and 10 children to protect. Moderate Hutus, including their prime minister, were being killed by Hutu extremists. The pastor correctly understood that discovery of his sheltering Tutsis would mean a death sentence for his family. Pastor Murinzi's situation included every factor that should activate a person's sociobiological systems: protective attachments to family members, peer affiliation with those in one's ethnic group, processes of kin recognition and social exchange that would relegate Tutsis to an outgroup status bearing few moral obligations. Yet Pastor Murinzi chose to hide the eight Tutsi women secretly, revealing their presence in his home only to two of his older children whom he trusted.

During the conflict, there was little food for the large household, so only table scraps could be diverted to the hidden women without revealing their presence. The women were barely surviving when French paratroopers entered the country 3 months after the genocide began and began setting up safe havens for Tutsi survivors. Pastor Murinzi managed to contact the French soldiers and planned the transport of the eight Tutsi women to safety.

How do we understand the exceptional strength of Pastor Murinzi's commitment to these Tutsi women? How do we understand the violence of Rwanda Christians against other Rwandan Christians? Nearly three-fourths of all Rwandans were Christians (Central Intelligence Agency, 2008). Both Tutsis and the Hutus who murdered them shared with Pastor Murinzi the same basic doctrines of Christian faith, love, and charity. Yet Tutsis who thought their churches might provide a safe haven were stabbed and dismembered as they tried to hide under the church pews.

Although we have no access to Pastor Murinzi's inner reflections, his conduct on the night that the women departed gives clues as to what mattered for him. On the night of their departure, he awakened the household at 2:00 A.M. He brought the eight women before his children. The children were shocked and confused, some fearing that the emaciated women were Tutsi ghosts who had come to haunt them. They were baffled as to how the women could have been living in their home for so long without their awareness. As they began to appreciate the reality of what they were witnessing, their father told them to take a good look at the women, reminding them "There, but for the grace of God, go any one of you. If you have a chance to help unfortunates like these ladies in times of trouble, make sure you do it—even if it means putting your own life at risk. This is how God wants us to live."

Immaculee Ilibagiza did not idealize Pastor Murinzi. At different times, she described him as ignorant, insensitive, and cruel. She struggled not to hate him after he refused to shelter her two brothers, who then were killed quickly by Hutu gangs. She resented his derogations of her father as a "bad Tutsi." Yet she also recognized that he placed his life and those of his wife and children at great risk by choosing to protect her. It was clear that Pastor Murinzi had an intense personal relationship with his God, with whom he spent daily time in prayer. This person–God relationship appeared to help him to focus on Immaculee as a person, not a category. This took priority over his Hutu allegiances or even his family relationships. Her category—Tutsi—was an aspect of who she was as a person; her person was not an aspect of her category.

Sociobiological Processes That Focus Outwardly

Sociobiological behavioral systems build secure boundaries around religious groups so that it is easy to determine who is a member of the group and who is not. This boundary around "us" and "we" regulates how freely information flows back and forth, usually limiting both the quantity and the kind of information about group members that outsiders can glean. Strong boundaries help religious groups to care for their own. Religious groups that thus thrive are participating in a larger evolutionary strategy of surviving by living within successful groups.

Peer affiliation and kin recognition serve major roles in maintaining religious group boundaries. Peer affiliation helps group members to feel a strong sense of solidarity with each other: "All for one and one for all." Kin recognition uses such markers as manner of talk, dress, or adherence to particular beliefs or rituals to discriminate who is inside and who is outside the group (Schneider, 2004, p. 397). Peer affiliation working the inside and kin recognition working the outside powerfully reinforce each other. Social exchange systems also play a role. Outsiders are likely to find that a different ethical ledger is used depending upon ingroup or outgroup status. Usually group members intuitively feel less accountable for responding in kind when outsiders perform good deeds but more likely to demand full reparations for any bad deeds.

Individual members of religious groups can benefit enormously when one's group is strong. Aside from specific religious content, they may receive better access to financial resources, a more desirable selection of mates, assistance with parenting, and protection from outside threats, to mention only a few potential benefits. Sociobiological systems work efficiently but mindlessly, though, without regard to any good larger than group survival and stability. A dark side to their operations can emerge, ranging from violence toward outsiders to deprivation of group members by virtue of lost access to resources from the outside world.

Kin Recognition

Other than maternal attachment, distinguishing who is and who is not "family" is perhaps the most essential of all social behaviors for animals in their struggles to survive. Even ants recognize who is kin and who isn't. Kin recognition is the heart of tribalism among humans. As such, it is a core element in the behavior of all religious groups. Human kin recognition mechanisms were biologically designed to detect physical resemblances, such as facial features, in order to recognize who is family and who is not (Kurland & Gaulin, 2005). Religious groups, however, can co-opt such bodily recognition systems by using other visible markers, such as using religious idioms in conversation, wearing distinctive dress, and making certain nonverbal religious signs in public settings. Such markers are fast and effective methods for separating ingroup and outgroups individuals.

Marc Galanter's (1999) account of his research within the Divine Light Mission cult illustrates both the fluidity and power of kin recognition processes in cohesive religious groups:

> The group's congeniality apparently extended to anyone designated as acceptable, as long as the proper signal was made. . . . We also saw the other side of the coin—how the group defined and protected its boundary between members and the outside world. . . . Our own status suddenly changed from inside to outside when a more suspicious member of the administrative group asked me if the project had been "approved" by senior figures from the Mission. In the absence of a definite response, our legitimacy was now open to question. Although it was not entirely clear what this approval entailed, a request was quickly relayed to the upper reaches of the Divine Light hierarchy and was then—to my surprise and distress— peremptorily turned down.
>
> The members I had met quickly withdrew their offers of friendship, providing an object lesson on exclusion from a cohesive group. I soon felt myself to be a nonperson, treated civilly but coolly, having become an out-

sider as rapidly as I had been made an insider. The very people who had hovered around us to help with our plans now found making conversation uncomfortable. People seemed to be looking *through* my colleague and me rather than at us.

Toward the end of the day approval came as suddenly as it had been withdrawn, with the information that a decision had been made at the "highest" level, presumably in consultation with the guru himself. Acceptance and offers of help came with rekindled warmth. As if automatically triggered, a renewed air of intimacy suffused our exchanges. (pp. 25–26)

Ingroups, Outgroups, and Social Identity

Kin recognition begins with a cognitive act: making a distinction between "us and we" and "them." This simple distinction sets a boundary around one's own people, separating an ingroup from other outgroups. To varying degrees of completeness, members of one's ingroup are felt emotionally in ways similar to blood kin, while outgroup members are felt as strangers. Distinguishing ingroup from outgroup usually activates closely associated sociobiological processes, particularly internalizing ones that create group solidarity: social hierarchy, peer affiliation, and social exchange.

Creating a boundary between ingroup and outgroups might seem to entail few consequences for how people in each group ought to be treated. However, ingroup membership is often wedded to social identity, which, in turn, sets the stage for stereotyping and stigmatizing that ultimately can prime exploitation or aggression toward outgroups (Kurzban & Leary, 2001). Social psychologist David Schneider (2004, p. 230) concluded in his review of social psychology research that "derogation of out-groups is one of the most fundamental and universal features of all societies and cultures."

Stereotyping and Stigmatization

Unlike many species, humans and other pack animals have social groups with flexible affiliative bonds that afford variable degrees for who is "one of us." In many species, mother–child attachments are the only strong affiliative relationships, and these may endure only briefly. However, humans routinely maintain multiple simultaneous group memberships, with some strong enough to imbue a sense of identity—"To these I belong. . . . This is who I am."

Social identity theorists (e.g., Tajfel, 1979, 1981, 1982) have articulated how social groups help establish a person's sense of identity. People make cognitive distinctions to distinguish who is in or out of their groups. They also reinforce perceived differences behaviorally by adopting "identity flags" as distinctive styles of speech or dress or other emblems. Language, particularly slang, is often used as a means of differentiation (Giles & Johnson, 1987).

The salience of identity with different groups ebbs and flows over time, depending on changing priorities, plans, and social situations. When in a particular social context, one group identity often matters more than another (Turner, 1987, 1991, 1999; Schneider, 2004). Marilyn Brewer (1991, 1993) has proposed that people in their groups try to balance two goals that are at risk for contradiction. They want to feel the surge in morale that comes from feeling similar, that "we are all the same." However, they also want to feel unique and special as individuals. One way to achieve both goals simultaneously is to derogate other groups. Jackson and Smith (1999) have studied this multi-determined model of social identity. They found both interdependency, the sense that the group's fate is one's own, and depersonalization, the sense that one is absorbed into the group so completely that members are more or less interchangeable, to play major roles in social identity. Individuals who feel insecure in their connection to or status within their group tend to rely more on depersonalization and interdependency. Such group members can be most at risk for demonizing those in other groups.

Strictly speaking, an intense identification with one's ingroup should not make hostility toward outgroups obligatory, except as a by-product of a wish to see one's ingroup in a positive light. Yet individuals and family clans in every culture claim their best human qualities, while disowning their worst by imputing them to outsiders. Perdue, Dovidio, Gurtman, and Tyler (1990) showed that even nonsense syllables resembling such words as "we," "our," and "us" were rated as more positive than syllables associated with the words "they," "them," and "their." Moreover, the ingroup words facilitated attribution of positive traits, while outgroup words facilitated attribution of negative traits. As a practical reality, there seems to be no "separate but equal."

William Graham Sumner (1907), a pioneer American sociologist, coined the term "ethnocentrism," to describe the tendency to view behavior as appropriate depending on one's own cultural standards while derogating other groups to the extent that they differ from one's ingroup. In similar vein to evolutionary psychologists of today, Sumner considered attachment to groups as necessary for human survival and division into competing groups as a natural part of social life. From this evolutionary perspective, conflict with other groups would not only heighten negative feelings toward the outgroups, but strengthen ingroup loyalties and feelings as well. *nothing like having an enemy to produce solidarity.*

Social Dominance: Status Hierarchies and Justification Ideologies

Pratto and Sidanius (Pratto, 1999; Sidanius & Prato, 1999) and Schneider (2004) have argued that all societies and cultures create status hierarchies and ideologies while privileging values that legitimate and conserve the existing hierarchy. Ethnocentrism and outgroup derogation thus exist within a broader *yes* context of social dominance.

Group hierarchies organized around age and gender appear to occur in all cultures. Those cultures that possess a surplus of food, goods, and other resources also develop hierarchies that can be set arbitrarily by distinctions about race, religion, ethnicity, and social class. The worst forms of group conflict and oppression are associated with these arbitrary-set hierarchies through racism, ethnocentrism, sexism, nationalism, classism, and regionalism.

Arbitrary-set hierarchies are typically supported by justification ideologies that are broadly disseminated within the culture. Justification ideologies are belief systems that produce derogatory stereotypes of those at the bottom of a social hierarchy and discriminatory beliefs about which abilities and attributes should be most valued (Pratto, 1999; Sidanius & Prato, 1999, Schneider, 2004). Such discriminatory beliefs and attitudes may even be shared by those who are victimized by them, thus weakening any claims for equality or justice. Justification ideologies legitimate existing hierarchies by producing power differentials among members of a society, while also using this power to create additional beliefs and institutional structures that perpetuate the power differentials.

Justification ideologies are the flywheels of prejudice. There are justification ideologies of different sorts. It has been estimated that right-wing authoritarianism and social dominance orientation together account for 40% of the variance for prejudice (Schneider, 2004). Authoritarianism emerges from a *NB.* social conservatism worldview centered upon vigilance against threats and dangers. Social dominance orientation, however, emerges from a worldview *yes* of economic conservatism that sees life in terms of competition and "survival of the fittest." Prejudice results when members of other groups are viewed as violating these values or as posing realistic or symbolic threats. Justification ideologies support the necessity of such worldviews for survival and well-being, both of societies and the individuals within them.

Religious beliefs and values serve important roles in either enhancing or attenuating group-based social inequalities (Sidanius & Pratto, 1999). They give credibility to social hierarchies and support negative attributions toward outgroups. Even when people are uncomfortable with the existence of a deprived underclass or the misery that stigma generates, they often tolerate stigma because they believe that the rejection, avoidance, and discrimination against stigmatized others is in some sense "right" (Crandall, 2000). Religious beliefs can serve as powerful justification ideologies that turn prejudice and stigma into acts of righteousness.

Social Exchange Typically Does Not Extend to Outgroup Members

Within one's group, generosity usually carries an unstated assumption of reciprocal altruism, expecting that one will receive generosity in return when in need. Such assumptions are typically not assumed for those in outgroups. No moral obligation may be felt to exist for the welfare of the stranger, and strangers by default are commonly experienced as potential perils. Even when religious people carry strong moral commitments, this aspect of sociobiology adds risk for dehumanization and aggression toward those in outgroups.

Religious kin recognition processes can create a moral conundrum, particularly when acting in concert with in-group peer affiliation and social exchange processes. Members of religious groups generally profess allegiance to the moral teachings of their religious tradition. Yet members of a religious group whose sacred scriptures teach brotherly love and compassion can instead, without irony or conflict, coerce, exploit, and murder those not belonging to their group.

Neurobiological Factors Amplify Religious Violence

As discussed in Chapter 2, neurobiological factors can interact with religious beliefs and ideologies to turn outgroup hostility into malignant violence. Social or psychological processes can trigger neurophysiological ones that, once initiated, begin operating autonomously, generating aggression that no longer is easily modulated by psychological or social factors. After brain threat systems lock in on an enemy, it is difficult to turn them back.

Religious language and beliefs can play potent roles in activating brain states of alarm. Religious leaders can use religious metaphors or speak with

scriptural authority to communicate that God has been dishonored, that outgroups are threatening, or that loyalty toward one's own religious clan demands
action. These attachment, kin recognition, and peer affiliation processes operate in all mammals to switch quickly between brain states of tranquility and
of alarm (Griffith & Griffith, 1994, pp. 66–68). These psychological or social
processes can deactivate brain circuits that underpin a person's ability to feel
empathy, to experience compassion, to reflect, and to engage in dialogue.
They can remove cortical top-down regulation of aggressive impulses (Stein,
2000). When these sociobiological processes dominate religious life, thinking
is replaced by the recitation of dogma, chanting of slogans, and mouthing of
moral sound bites. Religious beliefs that may have served in prior contexts as
guideposts of wisdom become instead little more than identity flags for who
is ingroup and outgroup. They no longer stimulate moral reflection or a quest
for spiritual truth.

Stigma Can Be Virtuous for Cults and Fundamentalist Religions

Cults and fundamentalist religious groups often seek stigmatization by the
mainstream culture. When a religious group wishes to keep a rigid boundary
with the outside secular world, stigma is an efficient mechanism for producing
it. Common sense might argue that shaved heads, long, flowing robes, chanting, and other odd, idiosyncratic behaviors would be aversive, particularly
when the religious group is already marginal within the larger society. The
evidence is to the contrary.

Galanter (1999, pp. 105–109) has studied how religious cults employ
boundary control to achieve a dual purpose of strengthening ingroup morale
and solidarity while keeping outsiders and their ideas at a distance. His studies
found that religious beliefs and behaviors were valued most when they cleanly
divided devout adherents from outsiders who viewed them as absurd or ridicu-
lous. In a study of the Divine Light Mission religious cult, Galanter (1978)
found "I am suspicious of nonmembers" to be the single item from a self-report
social cohesion scale that correlated highly with relief of emotional distress
when joining the group. Behaviors and attitudes of group members stigmatize outsiders, and these behaviors and attitudes are sufficiently hostile toward
outgroups that they, in turn, retaliate with stigma and prejudice against the
religious group. The two processes mutually reinforce each other.

In social psychology research, the cognitive efficiency of stigma appears
to be a major factor accounting for its endurance (Neuberg, Smith, & Asher,

2000). The "groupiness factor" is the extent to which stigma is based on membership in a definable group. By categorizing other people by a single identifiable mark, humans can quickly assume complex expectations for how members of that group are likely to perceive the world, to think, and to act (Miernat & Dovidio, 2000). Stigma exemplifies the philosophical concept of essentialism, which regards identification of membership in a particular category as the primary information needed about a person; that is, everyone in that category is presumed to share this primary essence (Miernat & Dovidio, 2000).

Certain religious groups are more likely to attract stigma than others. Groups with highly differentiated roles, functions, power, and status hierarchies have "high entitativity" and are most likely to be stigmatized within the broader culture. In such groups, members share common goals and have high levels of interaction with each other (Miernat & Dovidio, 2000). Cults and fundamentalist religious groups typically have high entitativity with their sharply defined boundaries, an authoritarian hierarchy of power and status, and intense interactions among group members that diminish their individuality. Galanter (1999) has similarly described charismatic groups with a strong emphasis upon shared beliefs, social cohesiveness, behavioral norms, and imputation of divine power to the group or its leadership. Such religious groups are likely to be stigmatized by outsiders, which becomes justification for their internal group structure and their vigilance and suspiciousness toward outsiders.

Dogmatic beliefs, unusual manners of dress, speech idioms, and high visible social practices are kin recognition markers that characterize nearly every cult or fundamentalist religious faith. The more exotic or nonmainstream the belief or dress, the better it functions for kin recognition and group boundary regulation (Galanter, 1999).

Religion Can Promote Guilt-Free Aggression

An array of social scientists and mental health clinicians have put forward evidence that "normal" people can commit inhumane acts despite the absence of a psychiatric illness (Lifton, 1986; Post, 2007). One need not have an antisocial personality disorder or paranoid psychosis in order to act brutally and cruelly. When group processes are intense, aggressive acts may need only the blessing of the group, usually put forward as behavioral expectations for "you are one of us" (Volkan, 2006). This blessing of the group can garner greater moral authority when the group is also a religious one and claims that the violence is, in fact, warranted by God.

Ryszard Kapuscinski (2006, p. 83) concluded from his international journalistic experiences that "the myths of many tribes and peoples include a belief that only we are human, the members of our clan, our society, and that Others—all Others—are subhuman, or not human at all." Settlers of the American West ventured forward in the manifest destiny belief that God was sending them forth. Little empathy or concern was expressed for the indigenous Native Americans who were killed in genocidal campaigns. When killing for God, one may even feel righteous or contemptuous of less zealous individuals who have qualms (Post, 2007). The social impact is profound. Individuals are motivated to find, even manufacture, religiously grounded justifications for violence. The religious call to action provides cover for moral accountability. The religiously violent can act out freely their darkest, most suppressed impulses to maim, to prey upon, to punish, to exact revenge, while feeling themselves only to be closer to God in the process.

Mental Health Clinicians Are Seldom First Responders

Aggression, coercion, stigmatization, and exploitation propelled by religions have produced some of the greatest moral catastrophes and humanitarian disasters that human beings have suffered. Religious justification ideologies have helped genocide, ethnic cleansings, racism, and abusive social hierarchies to thrive. As citizens and human beings, mental health clinicians have often wanted to join the battle against such human destruction. However, the ethical standards for mental health professionals largely preclude the aggressive use of intimidation and force often needed to stop violence in progress. Stopping religion-driven genocide is mainly a task for soldiers, police, attorneys, and policymakers. Skills for humanitarian relief in the aftermath of violence are to a great extent different from those possessed by most mental health professionals. Mental health clinicians are seldom offered first-responder roles where their professional skills can be utilized.

When mental health clinicians play a role in preventing religious violence, it is most often by promoting dialogue rather than debate and collaboration rather than polarization. Otherwise, mental health clinicians clean up after the fray, helping heal the emotionally wounded, treating symptoms, and rebuilding systems of health care. It is nevertheless useful to survey the scope of interventions to prevent religiously motivated violence in order to place in context the roles that mental health clinicians can play.

Psychosocial Interventions That Counter Harm from Sociobiological Religion

Some acts of religious violence are worldwide or societywide in scope, such as those by Al-Qaeda, antiabortion terrorists in the United States, Sikh fundamentalists in India, Jewish Gush Emunim extremists, Christian Aryan Nation ideologues, and the Aum Supreme Truth cult in Japan (Post, 2007). Others afflict only local communities. For example, a report on Calvary Temple, a Pentecostal church in Sterling, Virginia, appeared on the front page of *The Washington Post* after it was revealed that church leaders were using Biblical scriptures to order couples to terminate their marriage or parents to shun their children (Boorstein, 2008). The story focused on 16-year-old Rob Foster, who told his parents he no longer wanted to attend the church. Church leaders ordered the parents to throw Rob out of their home. They complied, telling their son that they would not see him or talk to him again, leaving him emotionally devastated. This church behavior has raised broad concerns among other churches and community social service agencies.

Interventions to counter such destructive uses of religion must be designed with sufficient sophistication to target the processes at work, often integrating the efforts of educational systems, news media, social service agencies, law enforcement, and political advocacy groups. Examination of three different types of interventional programs at the societal level displays principles that can also inform clinical interventions.

 Jerrold Post, counterterrorism political psychologist, has pointed out how religious terrorism is "bred in the bone" through early childhood education in radical religious institutions that equate violence with righteousness (Robins & Post, 1997; Post, 2007). Counterstrategies advocated by Post have targeted the management of information in the larger society and within terrorist groups rather than efforts to engage terrorists as individuals. For example, the Committee on the Psychological Roots of Terrorism for the 2005 Madrid Summit on Terrorism, Security and Democracy concluded that (Post, 2007, p. 4):

> Explanations at the level of individual psychology are insufficient in trying to understand why people become involved in terrorism. The concepts of abnormality or psychopathology are not useful in understanding terrorism. . . . Group, organizational, and social psychology, with a particular

emphasis on "collective identity," provides the most constructive framework for understanding terrorist psychology and behavior.

Such policies focus counter-terrorism efforts on strategic control of information operations (Post, 2007, p. 246):

1. Inhibiting potential terrorists from joining terrorist groups.
2. Producing dissension within terrorist groups.
3. Facilitating the exit of terrorists who choose to leave their groups.
4. Reducing material and political support for the group and its leader.
5. Insulating the target audience, the public, from the intended goals of the terrorist to terrorize.

Such a program would require resources of defense and intelligence agencies of national governments as well as support of nongovernment agencies that disseminate news and information within society.

Operating more locally, the Public Conversations Project is a program of conflict resolution that for two decades has worked to promote dialogue and to de-escalate conflict between pro-life and pro-choice advocates in the politicized abortion rights controversy (Chasin et al., 1996; Herzig & Chasin, 2006). In their interventions, the Public Conversations Project divides its attention between group processes and the personal engagement of individual pro-life and pro-choice advocates. Their general objective is to lead participants in politicized conflicts away from deadlock and toward authentic dialogue, in which responses are made to the other as a person, not a position. Their methods for creating contexts for dialogue have been drawn from clinical family therapy.

Guiding principles for the Public Conversations Project are illustrated in "dialogue dinners" involving both pro-life and pro-choice advocates. Participants must show at least a minimal degree of interest in understanding the perspectives of the other side. During the initial portion of the gathering, participants are not permitted to reveal their positions on abortion. Rather, they converse about each other's lives and make personal connections. After partaking dinner together, a structured conversation takes place in which each participant expresses his or her position on abortion issues, but does so in the context of critical personal life events that led them to that position. Participants thus situate their political commitments within their life stories. The Public Conversations Project dialogue dinners are structured to create a space for whole-person relatedness, empathy, and dialogue using group structures that inhibit kin recognition and peer affiliation behaviors.

A third type of intervention has focused primarily on engagement of religiously violent individuals rather than their groups. Narrative interview methods have been developed by Sara Cobb and colleagues for studying psychological processes that have fueled identity-based conflicts, ethnic cleansing, and genocide (Cobb, 2003). Cobb has examined perpetrators of human rights violations, such as the Rwanda genocide, who have been criminally convicted by the World Court at the Hague. Asking perpetrators why the violence occurred typically brings forth ideological justifications or dismissive responses. As an alternative, Cobb has utilized "ironic inquiry," which first seeks to understand what the perpetrators had been taught early in life about right and wrong and what their initial intentions were when they became politically involved. After this developmental narrative about moral values and commitments has been richly elaborated, it is juxtaposed with the consequences of the subsequent violence: "These were your original intentions. How was it that these were the consequences in the end?" This interview focuses upon the impacts of violence, its effects not only the victims but also on the humanity of the perpetrators and their family and community relationships.

Ironic inquiry has helped explicate how cultural myths and processes of meaning making have led to ethnic violence. Traditional legal and clinical interviews usually have built narrative accounts in which the perpetrator is seen as an evil, nonhuman character from whom others in society have little to learn. By contrast, Cobb's ironic inquiry has more often rehumanized the perpetrator and has produced links to the moral reasoning of everyday life, furthering our understanding for how "normal" people can commit horrific acts.

Post's antiterrorism program, the conflict resolution initiatives of the Public Conversations Project, and Cobb's use of ironic inquiry illustrate a range of methods used by social and political programs to counter destructive uses of ideology and religion. They illustrate the coupling of interventions that (1) block interactions solely driven by sociobiological agendas and (2) facilitate whole-person relatedness, empathy, compassion, and dialogue.

Mental health clinicians usually do not confront the worst excesses of religion-driven violence toward outgroups. However, they do face problems of externalized sociobiological religion when treating patients from cohesive religious groups or when seeking to protect a vulnerable member of a religious group. The issue then is how to conduct effective treatment despite one's outgroup status as a mental health professional. This requires effective management of any feelings of aversion toward the person, as religious countertransference, while extending whole-person relatedness, empathy, and compassion toward a religious group member who may not respond in kind (Griffith, 2006). Skills are needed that help clinicians and patients to experience each other as persons, not categories (Brewer & Miller, 1984, 1988; Griffith, 2010).

Advocating for Vulnerable Members of Religious Groups

Clinicians sometimes identify vulnerable members of religious groups who appear to be at risk for harm. Coercion, exploitation, and overt violence can present explicitly in cases of domestic violence or child abuse. Other problems are less dire but involve suffering produced in part by religious beliefs, practices, or mandated social roles.

Mr. Milner, for example, was a 50-year-old man for whom psychiatric consultation had been requested because of concerns regarding his rage toward his teenage daughter when he discovered she was in a sexual relationship with a boy, a violation of the values of his fundamentalist Christian faith. Mr. Milner reluctantly agreed to the consultation only after strong urgings from his primary care physician. The interview was conducted by a psychiatry resident whom I was supervising.

Mr. Milner looked at the resident skeptically. After a brief discussion of the purpose for the consultation, the resident asked, "Do you have any important beliefs I should be aware of?"

"I was born and raised in the Church of God," Mr. Milner responded. "I have never doubted what I was taught and will be a devout Christian forever." He then began talking angrily about his daughter's deception in keeping the sexual relationship hidden. He felt betrayed and found it difficult not to banish her from his household.

Before moving discussion to Mr. Milner's daughter, the resident inquired again about Mr. Milner's faith: "Would you tell me more about your family's values?"

"Of course," Mr. Milner responded. "I believe that sex before marriage is a sin, but if the person is an adult they have to make that decision on their own. Teenagers should not have sex at all because they lack responsibility. If you do have a sexually active child, the parents need to deal with it. This is the part I'm having trouble with. I don't know how to deal with it. I find it almost impossible to not think of her as evil, even though she is my daughter."

By this point, Mr. Milner's countenance had softened. The resident asked Mr. Milner for a more detailed account of what had happened. Mr. Milner teared during the telling. The resident acknowledged how this was an awful dilemma in which Mr. Milner was caught between his commitment to his God and church and his love for his daughter. Guessing that there was also a larger context for the dilemma, he asked, "If you were to change your belief for the sake of your daughter, what would happen?"

"Well, first of all, I'm not sure I can change my belief," Mr. Milner stated. "But if I could, my entire church would probably ostracize me. I think my wife would be the only person who would support me."

This explanation helped clarify the breadth of his dilemma. Mr. Milner's struggle involved more than his personal religious beliefs. His response was a loyalty test within his church community. It was clear that there were practical consequences at stake, not just an abstract theological debate. He felt torn between the available choices. The psychiatry resident was then able to facilitate Mr. Milner meeting with a trusted church elder, who could provide counsel and support from the church leadership in finding ways to parent his daughter short of extruding her from her family and church.

From his own perspective, the resident was an advocate for the daughter and wanted to preserve her relationship with her father. His concern in the interview, however, was to establish sufficient relatedness with a reluctant Mr. Milner so that further conversation might continue. This required grasping the father's cognitive and emotional perspectives, while avoiding any hint of threat that might prompt his withdrawal. The resident began by inquiring about, acknowledging, and conveying respect for Mr. Milner's religious identity. He could feel empathy, rather than judgment, for Mr. Milner by clarifying quickly the role of Mr. Milner's religious community as a "church family" that was vigorous both in the support it provided to its members and in its expectations for their fealty in return. Grasping how Mr. Milner was caught in pincers between heartfelt attachment to his daughter and a high-entitativity religious community helped dissipate the disdain the resident felt initially toward a father who would consider disowning his child for the sake of religious faith.

The Tenuous Position of an Outgroup Clinician

A clinical strategy for countering religiously promoted aggression or neglect toward others is generally two-pronged: first, to avoid interactions that would trigger further escalation of defensive sociobiological behaviors, such as more intensive boundary monitoring, dominance–submission behaviors, or ingroup solidarity; and second, to locate and focus on aspects of religious life that represent the patient's personal spirituality. The aim of intervention is a relative strengthening of personal spirituality as it influences the patient's religious life.

This strategy can be difficult to implement when a clinician is in the ambivalently held, provisional status of an outgroup member. A clinician must stay mindful of the limitations of one's outgroup status. Needed conversations may not be welcomed. The most potent intervention can be to model within the clinical encounter the whole-person relatedness, empathy, respect, and compassion that may be absent from the patient's behavior because of the strictures of defensive sociobiology.

Externalizing sociobiological processes most often present as difficulties in establishing a therapeutic alliance or as precipitous disruptions in treatment. Mental health clinicians, and psychiatrists in particular, are sometimes stigmatized by religious fundamentalists as practitioners of evil arts. Under these conditions, it can seem nearly impossible to build a therapeutic alliance that is sufficient to support treatment.

For example, I was asked by Ms. Bass's internist to evaluate whether she needed psychiatric treatment for depression. Ms. Bass was hospitalized because of a rheumatological disorder. Her recovery appeared to be hindered by her grief from the recent death of her mother. She had been withdrawn, apathetic, and minimally participative in her physical rehabilitation program.

Ms. Bass was curled up in bed with a sheet over her head when I entered the room. I apologized for awakening her and explained her medical team's concerns and their request that I meet with her. I let her know that they had told me about her mother's death. I asked whether she had been able to sleep the night before. "No," she said, beginning to weep inconsolably. I asked whether her mother's death had been expected or unexpected. She said that her mother had been chronically ill with leukemia and was then diagnosed with a worrisome infection, but her death from a sudden heart attack was an unexpected shock. "She was my best friend," she sobbed. I asked how she coped during a time like this. "I ask God," she said. I wanted to learn more about her religious faith in order to understand better how we might respond to her needs. I also wanted to clarify whether her suffering was normal bereavement or whether she might have a depressed mood that needed psychiatric treatment, as was the opinion of her medical team.

"Do you sense that God hears your prayer?" I asked.

"I pray for him to lift my burden," she responded.

"What do you ask God?" I asked.

"There are two kinds of prayers," she said, "One in tongues and the other in my language."

"Which prayer brings more comfort?" I asked.

"They both do," she said.

Then she looked at me sharply and asked in an accusatory tone, "Do you believe in God?"

I could tell that she was freshly aware that I was a psychiatrist. I realized that her question was one intended to discern whether she could safely speak with openness. I was unsure what meaning would be given either a "yes" or "no" response. I had no way of knowing what she meant by either "God" or "belief in God." As a default, I spoke from that which I could feel authentically. I nodded and responded, "I believe what you are telling me, that you ask God to lift your burden, and you do feel him lift your burden."

My response did not pass the test. "But do you believe in God?" she asked again.

"Yes," I said, responding as best I could with honesty, while realizing I could not understand the horizons of meaning these words held for her.

I tried to shift the topic back from my identity to her well-being as the clinical question of concern, realizing that this still might not allay her distrust. "It sounds like God is your greatest support in a time like this." I said. "Are there ways that the doctors and nurses here are also helpful?"

"There are some nurses who know me because I'm been here a lot of times. They help me," she responded.

I asked about the ways that the nurses were helpful, and she told about some specific incidents when nurses were sensitive or thoughtful to her.

She declined a subsequent question about the loss of her mother, stating that she didn't want to talk to speak more about it. Gauging that I had reached the comfort limits of her personal openness, I shifted the interview away from her experience and toward a more factual inquiry about her medical care: her symptoms, medications, and plans for outpatient care. I told her that I would talk with the nurses and her doctors and that we would continue to try to help her.

Ms. Bass's question, "Do you believe in God?," posed a challenge for my psychiatric interview. In a formal psychotherapy, I might have responded, "Can I ask first—Are you concerned I may not be able to understand you? Or that I might not respect your faith?" As Karen Armstrong has noted, the statement: "I believe in God" has no meaning outside a specific context, spoken by a specific person (Armstrong, 1993). However, Ms. Bass had not asked to meet with me in the first place, and such a response likely would have amplified her wariness by its intrusiveness. Her question seemed to ask that I declare whether I was in her trusted group, so my response was simply, "Yes." Afterward, I made an additional response when her wariness persisted—I shifted the interview away from further conversation about her experience of her God. My guiding principle was not to force conversation that would compel her to demand a declaration of "friend or enemy" unless there were important and overriding ethical or clinical reasons to do so. Here, there were not. In her grief, she belonged in her own community, and I was not a part of it.

Understanding constraints on the treatment relationship from religious stigmatization can help a clinician best position him- or herself to be therapeutically useful. It is necessary to accept one's otherness and outgroup status, which means assertively avoiding behaviors or communications that prompt defensive (sociobiological) responses.

Commitment to Whole-Person Relatedness Helps Quiet Defensive Sociobiology

As an outgroup member, a clinician often has limited influence with members of cohesive religious groups. A respectful but persistent whole-person relatedness extended toward a patient with rigid group boundaries is perhaps the most potent of clinical interventions. Responding to another person as someone capable of reflection, empathy, concern, and compassion tends to recruit the same processes within the other person, while tempering activation of defensive sociobiological systems.

This kind of whole-person relatedness is akin to the therapeutic posture that good psychodynamic psychotherapists have always tried to offer their patients: an empathic and compassionate understanding that transcends any social category or categorization of likableness. However, traditional psychotherapy has never achieved much success in addressing patients' problems when they have been embedded in powerful families or social groups whose roles, hierarchies, and boundary regulation devalue the expertise of mental health clinicians, keeping them at an emotional, and often physical, distance.

Mental health clinicians too often have been regarded as godless and thereby viewed with suspiciousness or overt hostility.

What psychodynamic formulations have often lacked has been a complex understanding of the social processes of stigma. The therapeutic power of psychodynamic psychotherapy rests in its capacity for understanding a person as an individual. It draws its data primarily from dialogue with an individual about his or her perceptions, thoughts, feelings, and actions. Family, cultural, and social contexts of clinical problems are often only sketchily considered. A patient in a cohesive religious or ideological group, however, is operating primarily within a group identity, not an individual one. The patient presents as a socially determined sociobiological self, not a personal self. The patient presents as a role or a position, not as a person. Clinical data for understanding the patient are more likely to be found in the study of the social structure and communicational processes of the patient's group rather than an analysis of the patient's psyche as an individual. A clinician lacking a nuanced understanding of this social context is left unfocused and without interventions that have an impact.

Irving Yalom's story "The Fat Lady" provides a vivid account for how stigma can be addressed in a traditional psychodynamic psychotherapy (Yalom, 1989). Yalom's psychotherapy with Betty, a morbidly obese woman, illustrates both similarities and differences between traditional psychotherapy and a clinical posture oriented toward sociobiological and neurobiological contexts. In his moving account, Yalom reveals with courage and honesty his long-running personal struggle with stigmatizing fat people, acknowledging that "I have always been repelled by fat women. I find them disgusting" (p. 88). Confronting his own stigma-driven prejudice was a core element of the psychotherapy's success. After reflection, he located its origins in his unhappiness with early life relationships involving his mother and other obese parenting figures, the meaning obesity took on for him as a marker of first-generation immigrant families, and the ostracization of overweight kids in his elementary school.

Yalom struggled in his efforts to listen and attend to Betty, feeling bored, glancing at the clock, and mindlessly waiting for their sessions to end. As the story proceeded, however, Betty transformed gradually from a shallow, dull, one-dimensional person to a richly complex, interesting, and likable human being. This transformation happened as Yalom steadily confronted his prejudice, dealt with it, and began seeing Betty as a unique and potentially interesting person.

Yalom brought to his psychotherapy with Betty a commitment "to stand by that person: to spend all the time and all the energy that proves necessary for the patient's improvement; and most of all, to relate to the patient in an intimate, authentic manner" (Yalom, 1989, p. 91). He also brought a sense of professionalism that he was responsible for managing his countertransference responses as irrational thoughts and feelings that originated out of his own early life learning. Yalom's psychotherapy with Betty was a success in that she lost weight, which lessened the stigma she faced, while also recovering a sense of herself as a competent, desirable person. By the end of the therapy, Betty was able to speak directly with Yalom about her awareness since the beginning of the therapy that her appearance was repulsive to others. Moreover, she acknowledged her own self-disgust and the disgust she felt at the sight of other obese people. The therapy ended with mutual openness, respect, and emotional intimacy between Yalom and Betty.

Why was Irving Yalom's psychotherapy with Betty so successful when psychodynamic psychotherapy generally has not been so with stigma-affected religious patients such as Mr. Burns in Chapter 7? The issue appears to have more to do with what psychodynamic psychotherapy has failed to do rather than with what it has done with consistent effectiveness. As with Irving Yalom, psychodynamic psychotherapists are steadfast in their commitment to understand a patient as an individual. However, they have been generally less interested in understanding the structure of the social and relational world within which a patient lives. From the start, Betty brought to Yalom a determined individuality. Mr. Burns did not offer this. When a patient's identity, both psychologically and ideologically, is wedded to the group, not to a sense of oneself as an individual, then psychodynamic psychotherapists struggle. A more even-handed approach can be suggested that balances attentiveness to "patient as person" with attentiveness to "patient as family member" or "patient as group member." A sociobiological and neurobiological perspective adds to a psychodynamic perspective a framework for understanding the workings of social identity, social dominance, and boundary regulation within groups whose members may have less of a personal self than a group-regulated sociobiological self.

Avoiding Activation
of Defensive Boundary Regulation

Successful management of felt aversion toward religious patients is a first priority. Religious countertransference refers to the negative emotions and hostile impulses triggered by language, manner of dress, or attitudes of religious patients who are hostile or rejecting toward clinicians (Griffith, 2006). Stigma calls out for counterstigma. When a clinician feels extruded and stigmatized by a religious group whose identity flags are not shared, a natural emotional response is to counterstigmatize. Religious patients acting in ways that are hostile, dismissive, or condescending are easily viewed by clinicians as bizarre or "crazy." Empathy is difficult, and scapegoating and ridicule come easily.

A deliberate focus upon courtesy and etiquette is a first step toward managing religious countertransference. Showing respectful interest in a patient's religious identity is a "cultural handshake" that conveys safety. One hopes that a patient can experience the clinical encounter as a neutral zone in which there will be no threats, thus permitting a relaxation of defenses. The FICA interviewing tool is commonly used by primary care physicians who are interested in incorporating spirituality into patient care (George Washington Institute for Spirituality and Health, 2008). It provides an example of such a cultural handshake:

F— Faith and belief ("Do you consider yourself to be spiritual or religious? Do you have spiritual beliefs that help you cope with stress?")

I— Importance ("What importance does your faith or belief have in your life?")

C—Community ("Are you part of a spiritual or religious community?")

A—Address in care ("How would you like me, your health care provider, to address these issues in your health care?")

A clinician's initial aim is to learn enough about the patient's identity to be able to convey respect. The FICA questions or similar ones can go a long distance toward an understanding that enables a physician to interact respectfully, as illustrated by the psychiatry resident's first question to Mr. Milner: "Do you have any important beliefs I should be aware of?"

Although counterintuitive, discovery of differences in beliefs and worldview often advances mutual respect more than discovery of shared commonalities, provided that the inquiry is conducted from authentic interest and that discovered differences are treated with respect (Levinas, 1961). A person who feels vulnerable can best relax defenses when it is clear that the other understands one's uniqueness and identity.

Openness for dialogue is often signaled more nonverbally than verbally, by the meeting of gaze, deepened breathing, and relaxation of muscles. Verbally, questions then draw more open and elaborate responses free of debate. Successful conveyance of respect helps open the possibility of conversation. The vignettes about Ms. Bridges in Chapter 7 and Mr. Chin in the Introduction and revisited in Chapter 7 illustrated how this could be achieved. The prior vignette about Ms. Bass, however, showed how this sometimes is unachievable. It is then best not to attempt to force dialogue when its preconditions are absent. One can then ask with whom else the patient could possibly meet in dialogue, if not with oneself. This was the case with April, in Chapter 5. The conversation with Mr. Burns, in Chapter 7, ended with a similar suggestion.

Using a Sociobiological Perspective to Help Manage Religious Countertransference

A sociobiological perspective helps grasp complexities in a clinician's reflexive aversion toward a religiously determined patient who is aggressive or dismissive, enabling more nuanced responses. A clinician can feel stereotyped, stigmatized, and denigrated when a religiously determined patient uses kin recognition and peer affiliation processes to set boundaries the clinician cannot cross. Hostility and disdain, as countertransferential feelings, can be difficult to push off to the side. As with Mr. Burns, it can prove more fruitful to formulate how the patient's sociobiological religiousness is generating cognitive and emotional perspectives that drive the hostility. Such a formulation can make negative affects more manageable. Cognitive and emotional perspective taking are essential prerequisites for empathy.

Four guidelines can aid a clinician:

1. *Focus on the person, not the category.* It is critical that a clinician relate to the patient as someone larger and more complex than self-proclaimed categories, even though the patient may ask to be regarded only as a born-again Christian or a Muslim or a Jew.

2. *Focus on the patient's otherness as a person.* The clinician's attitude can convey interest in a patient's aspects that are not yet known or understood, even when he or she insists there is nothing more that needs knowing and when it is tempting to believe that to be the case. Relating to a patient as someone still to be known helps attenuate countertransferential feelings.

3. *Do not take personally what, in fact, is not personal.* A religious patient's judgment that a clinician is unfit for conversation generally is based on perceived identity flags that mark the clinician as a member of a distrusted group, hardly an assessment of the clinician's personhood;

4. *Aim to parry, not to win.* A clinician must avoid being redefined in his or her identity by the patient's sociobiological specifications. The trick is to refuse submission to a patient's aggressive moves without retaliating, which predictably would elevate further the patient's defensiveness. The aim is not to win an argument with cleverness but to refuse objectification by the patient. Holding the high ground means sticking with a stance of whole-person relatedness despite provocations to the contrary. This often succeeds over time. By persistently relating as a subject, not as an object, the possibility of future dialogue is preserved.

It helps to stay mindful of Levinas's (1961) proposal that it is through encounters with those who in their otherness stand outside our familiar worlds that our own personhood is revealed to us. We thus need to know the other who comes as a stranger. As a mental health clinician, a fundamentalist religious group member who stigmatizes me is my Other to know. This awareness helps me to value rather than to dread such encounters.

III

✦

WHEN MENTAL ILLNESS
INFILTRATES RELIGIOUS LIFE

RELIGIOUS LIFE SHOULD EXPRESS THE WHOLENESS OF A person's being. An active psychiatric disorder, however, can rob a person of a capacity to speak, feel, or act fully as a person. Dysfunctional brain circuits instead can cripple accurate processing of information. Hallucinations, confused or delusional thinking, anxious preoccupations, or overwhelming mood states can dominate and distort religious experience. In some cases, processes essential to personal spirituality—dialogue, self-reflection, empathy—may simply fail to operate. Psychiatric illness can malform religious experience, amplify suffering in daily life, and create caricatures of spirituality. Assessing impacts of mental illness in religious life is a clinical challenge, however. Intense religious experiences, particularly in group contexts, can produce within a normal person literally any symptom of psychiatric illness, including hallucinations, delusional fears, dissociative trance states, or panic anxiety. Such a person is badly served by a label of mental illness. Moreover, a person with a bonafide mental illness may yet be able to elaborate a rich, complex spiritual life, in which personal spirituality helps provide resilience against the illness. A mentally ill person can have a normal religious life. Treatment of psychiatric illness comingled with religious experience is daunting but vital in its importance. For many patients, effective psychiatric treatment that controls hallucinations, delusional thinking, anxiety, depression, mania, or dissociation tempers suffering, enlivens daily existence, and opens fresh possibilities for relatedness both with the Divine and with other people.

181

9

✦

Religion That Is a Voice
for Mental Illness

MIDMORNING ON JUNE 20, 2001, RUSTY YATES, A NASA FLIGHT engineer in Houston, Texas, received a terrifying call from his wife, Andrea. "You need to come home," she said.

"What's going on?" Rusty asked.

"You need to come home. It's time. I did it," Andrea responded.

Worried, Rusty asked Andrea to explain, but she only said, "It's the children."

"Which one?" Rusty asked.

"All of them," Andrea responded.

Rusty rushed home, but police and ambulances were already there and prevented him from entering. He collapsed on the lawn when told that all his five children were dead. Andrea had drowned each child and then called the police to tell them that she was a bad mother and should be punished (Ramsland, 2005). The police found the bodies of the four youngest children laid out on a bed, clothed and still wet. The body of the fifth, the oldest son, was still submerged in the bathtub.

Andrea Yates, from a family with a history of mental illnesses, had suffered from recurrent postpartum depression. After the killings of her children, psychiatric evaluations found her to have a major depressive disorder with psychotic features. In her delusional thinking, she believed that Satan had already won the battle for her soul (Sweetingham, 2006). She believed that killing her children while they were still younger than the "age of accountability" meant that their souls would live with God in heaven. She also believed that upon her execution for the murders, Satan would be slain together with her. Forensic psychiatrist Phillip Resnik testified that "it is my opinion, with medical certainty, that Mrs. Yates on June 20, 2001, believed she was doing what was right for the children" (Sweetingham, 2006). Her medical records showed that her psychiatrist, during prior weeks, had been concerned about her worsening symptoms and had been raising the dosages of her antidepressant medications in response. Nevertheless, a Texas jury rejected Andrea Yates's insanity defense, convicted her of murder, and sentenced her to life imprisonment with eligibility for parole in 40 years. The sentence was subsequently reversed in a second jury trial, and Yates was eventually committed to a state mental hospital with a verdict of not guilty by reason of insanity (Associated Press, 2006).

Andrea Yates's tragedy was more complex than could be accounted for solely by psychiatric diagnoses of major depressive disorder and postpartum psychosis. The Yates family also had been long immersed within a fundamentalist Christian religious cult whose beliefs had been incorporated into Andrea Yates's delusional thinking.

For 9 years the Yates family had been disciples of Michael Woroniecki, an itinerant, self-ordained, "fire-and-brimstone" preacher. Woroniecki preached that mainstream Christian churches spoke for the Antichrist and had promulgated a "false and polluted twentieth century gospel" that held no redemptive power. He believed that education was a sin, working was part of the curse placed by God on Adam and Eve, and Christ's disciples must live a jobless life preaching the Christian gospel as prophets. He proclaimed that children of those not adherent to this discipline would be destined for hell. A 1995 video watched by Andrea Yates taught that children were not accountable until 12 years old, the "age of accountability," and that babies were better off aborted than to grow up with parents who were "witches and wimps" and who would doom their children to hellfire (Wikipedia, 2006). Woroniecki regarded women, particularly those who worked outside the home, as "witches" and "daughters of Eve" who were genetically rebellious against God's creation, and men who submitted to women were "wimps." The 1995 video taught that it was better for parents to commit suicide than to cause their children to be damned. Two months after hearing the Woroniecki message, Andrea Yates was twice hospitalized for suicide attempts.

The Woroniecki teachings also had shaped Rusty Yates's behavior as a husband and father. Andrea's psychiatrist had warned the Yates that having more children would ensure future episodes of psychotic depression (Wikipedia, 2006). Yet her husband decided that they should follow Woro... admonition to have as many children as God should grant them. Andrea submitted to his decision in accordance with the Woroniecki teaching that a wife must submit to her husband lest she become a "contentious witch," like Eve in the Garden of Eden. In the days before the killings, Andrea's psychiatrist had stressed to the couple the importance of Andrea not being left alone with the children at home. Yet the weekend before the killings Rusty told family members that he would leave Andrea home alone for an hour twice a day so that she would not become overly dependent upon him and his mother for taking care of her maternal responsibilities.

Andrea Yates's killing of her children was a product both of a psychotically deranged mind and the beliefs and practices of a religious cult. Interaction between the two was necessary in order for the killings to have occurred. Psychiatric illnesses do not operate in a vacuum. Their contents reflect the ideas of the surrounding culture, including religious culture. Intense emotions evoked by religion can provoke relapse of a psychotic illness. The Woroniecki religious group displayed to a powerful degree sociobiological processes that produced an extreme hierarchy of power and suppression of any individuality of Andrea Yates as a person. At the same time, her psychosis grotesquely amplified the power of these beliefs and practices.

How Psychiatric Illness Matters

Psychiatric illness represents a failure of information processing in the brain that distorts a person's experience of life's events and circumstances. It often exaggerates the intensity of suffering. When stressed by adversity, a person normally may feel demoralized, in shock, grief stricken, or humiliated, depending on the kind of adversity (see Figure 9.1). In vulnerable individuals, however, these normal responses of suffering can secondarily trigger onset of

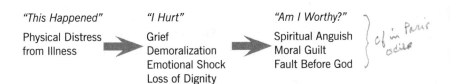

"This Happened"	"I Hurt"	"Am I Worthy?"
Physical Distress from Illness	Grief Demoralization Emotional Shock Loss of Dignity	Spiritual Anguish Moral Guilt Fault Before God

FIGURE 9.1. Spirituality is a normal response to the experience of living. Neither adversity nor the experience of it necessarily produces a spiritual crisis, but a spiritual quest is a common human response in coping.

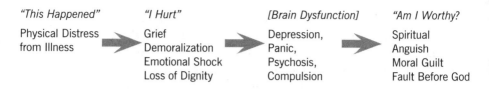

"This Happened"	*"I Hurt"*	*[Brain Dysfunction]*	*"Am I Worthy?*
Physical Distress from Illness	Grief Demoralization Emotional Shock Loss of Dignity	Depression, Panic, Psychosis, Compulsion	Spiritual Anguish Moral Guilt Fault Before God

FIGURE 9.2. Psychiatric illness represents a system failure of information processing within the nervous system. It amplifies suffering and distorts the meaning of experience. The spiritual quest that ensues may proceed in response to malformed experience, with consequent distortions of meaning that risk harm to self or others.

an anxiety, mood, psychotic, or dissociative disorder. Such psychiatric disorders distort how life experiences are interpreted, sometimes confuse thinking, and often magnify the severity of the original suffering (see Figure 9.2). A psychiatrically ill person who then invokes religion or spirituality to cope is responding to a distorted image of the adverse life event, not to an accurate representation. The psychiatrically ill person is dealt an unfair hand.

For clinicians, there are two questions of overriding concern when suggestive signs indicate that psychiatric illness may play a role in destructive uses of religion:

1. Should the disturbing religious behavior be regarded primarily as a symptom of mental illness?
2. If so, can psychiatric treatment, particularly psychopharmacological treatments, attenuate the disturbing behavior?

Answering these questions can be a difficult challenge. As the Yates's tragic story demonstrated, destructive religious behavior rarely is a pure product of psychiatric illness. In nearly all cases, a complex interaction must occur between a person's psychiatrically ill brain and the family, social, and cultural factors promoting the harmful behavior.

Psychiatric Disorders Emanate from Brain Dysfunction

Serious psychiatric disorders—depression, mania, anxiety, psychosis, dissociation—represent dysfunction in major brain systems that process information. A general paradigm has emerged in the latter 20th century that now explains most major psychiatric disorders in terms of dysfunctional regulation of subcortical systems by executive systems of the prefrontal cortex. The prefrontal cortex, which constitutes nearly one-fourth of the human brain, operates in much the same manner as an executive program in a computer that manages the time sharing of all other programs and regulates interactions among other computers. The prefrontal cortex conducts this executive role with close support of the hippocampus and dorsal cingulate gyrus, which help manage memory and distribution of the brain's attentional resources, respectively. Two other subcortical systems organize behavioral responses to emotionally salient events, generating emotions that motivate a person either to move toward (gratification seeking) or away from (threat avoiding) stimuli in the environment. The brain's reward system is centered in the ventral striatum (the moving toward). The threat avoidance system is centered in the amygdala and insula (the moving away). When the brain operates at its best, the ventral striatum and amygdala/insula each generate their particular emotional responses, and adjustments by the prefrontal cortex keep their influences at levels appropriate for achieving long-term life goals. Toward these ends, the hippocampus and dorsal cingulate gyrus keep attention properly focused. They serve as the brain's "spotlight" that stays trained upon long-term priorities of the prefrontal cortex.

All anxiety disorders are characterized by an amygdala that is metabolically hyperactive. This hyperactive amygdala can override its regulation from the prefrontal cortex. Depression is similarly characterized by an amygdala that is hyperactive as well as a ventral striatum that is underactive, both of which escape regulation by the prefrontal cortex. Psychotic disorders arise from fundamental design problems within the prefrontal cortex itself such that working memory is impaired in its ability to take brief "mental snapshots" of the world to support processes of reasoning. As a result, a patient with schizophrenia has what National Institute of Mental Health psychiatric researcher Daniel Weinberger has described as a "noisy brain." In schizophrenia, instability of working memory secondarily produces all manner of faulty percepts and aberrant reasoning. As a result, executive functions such as prioritizing, judging, and planning are impaired, and delusions and hallucinations confuse thinking.

Sociobiological systems mediate interactions between a patient's interpersonal world and his or her brain. These interactions can activate psychiatric symptoms when they stress vulnerable brain systems. In turn, disordered information from a dysfunctional brain is reflected in a person's relational and social world via the different sociobiological systems.

Distinguishing Psychiatric Symptoms
from Troubling, but Normal, Religious Behaviors

Distinguishing symptoms of psychiatric disorders from the breadth of thoughts, emotions, and behaviors capable of expression by a non-ill religious person can be difficult. There is no foolproof formula for distinguishing psychiatric illness from odd or idiosyncratic behaviors that can be produced during religious experience by a non-ill person. There are no laboratory test that can be conducted. There is no specific symptom whose presence is a sure marker for psychiatric illness. Hallucinations, delusional fears, dissociative trance states, and panic anxiety can occur among otherwise normal people during intense religious experiences.

However, there are clues as to what lies within the range of normality and what is psychopathological. Behaviors resulting from the distorted information processing of a psychiatric illness are often outside the range of normality in terms of activation threshold, duration, intensity, and modulation (Horwitz & Wakefield, 2007). Behaviors in response to stressors are either inappropriate in character or disproportionate in severity. For example, bereavement is a normal emotional response to loss of a vital relationship. However, intense bereavement after loss of a mere acquaintance (too low a threshold) or absence of bereavement after the death of a family member (too high a threshold) may suggest a psychiatric disorder. Likewise, rage that comes too easily, too intensely, endures too long, or is unremitting even after a provoking event has ended may suggest psychiatric illness. The despair and self-condemnation of Andrea Yates were notable for their severity, pervasiveness, and failure to respond to any measures of spiritual comfort. For Andrea Yates, these factors favored a diagnosis of major depressive disorder rather than a difficult adjustment to the stress of a new baby.

Abnormal forms of cognition also serve as clues to a psychiatric diagnosis. The key is not so much the specific content of a patient's thoughts but rather how the thinking is structured. Abnormal forms include disjunctures of logic in the smooth flow of thoughts, an absence of awareness for other people's thoughts or feelings, and nonmodulated thoughts or emotions that dominate a patient's mental life to excess. For example, the psychotic thought that often characterizes schizophrenia cannot sustain a smooth, logical flow of ideas. The associative links between the words of schizophrenic thought are often odd, bizarre, or illogical (loose associations), whereas the rapid flow of manic thought shows each new idea veering off in a new direction so that the point of the conversation is lost (flight of ideas). Commonly, psychotic thought is characterized by paranoia, meaning that emotional appraisal and logic are unable to determine who is trustworthy, so the person retreats to a defensive posture of pervasive suspiciousness and excessive vigilance for potential threats. Severe mental illnesses are commonly characterized by impaired perspective taking, so that a patient is literally unable to imagine how other people might think or feel about a situation and has no access to common wisdom for what makes sense. Such disturbances in form of thinking can indicate an underlying psychiatric illness that is shaping a person's experiences and, in essence, hijacking religious life.

Psychiatric illnesses are also associated with other co-occurring symptoms. Major depression and mania are usually associated with disturbances in sleep, energy, hedonia, appetite, and libido in addition to the elevated or depressed mood that may be the presenting concern. Schizophrenia and other psychoses are usually associated with disorganized thinking, apathy, impaired sociality, and difficulties with such executive functions as planning, organizing, and multitasking.

Finally, disturbing behaviors that are largely shaped by psychiatric illness often remit to dramatic degrees when treated with appropriate psychiatric medications. Disturbing behaviors generated by normal sociobiological systems rarely respond to psychiatric medications. Normal grief, demoralization, and stigma-induced humiliation, although productive of suffering, do not benefit from treatment with antidepressant medications. Mood-stabilizing and antipsychotic medications have no benefits for the up-and-down mood shifts or frazzled thinking that life stresses produce among people without underlying psychiatric illnesses. Even so, response to medication itself is not a perfect test for psychiatric illness. Benzodiazepines (diazepam, alprazolam, lorazepam) and alcohol will help anyone feel more relaxed, not just those with anxiety disorders. Psychostimulants, such as methylphenidate or amphetamine, will sharpen any person's concentration, not just those with attention-deficit disorder. Despite these limitations, a clear-cut response to medication nevertheless is an additional piece of evidence that can be weighed when combined with other dimensions of assessment.

Clinical assessment for distinguishing idiosyncratic but normal religious behavior from psychiatric illness must thus include a number of questions:

1. Could a disturbing behavior plausibly represent the normal behavioral response of a sociobiological system? Examples include grief from losses, demoralization from overwhelming circumstances, emotional shock from unexpected traumatic events, and humiliation from loss of dignity.
2. Is the intensity of the behavior proportional to the initiating event?

3. Does the behavior remit if the stressors that initiated it are terminated?
4. Are there associated symptoms of a psychiatric disorder?
5. Are there identifiable biological or psychosocial risk factors for occurrence of a psychiatric disorder?
6. Is there a history of a psychiatric disorder? If so, has it shown a pattern of relapse and recurrence?
7. Is there a robust response to a psychiatric medication? If not, can the failure of response be attributed to psychological or social stressors that are so overwhelming that any beneficial effects of medication would be overridden?

For Andrea Yates, the severity of her depression, its persistence, and its associated apathy, disorganization of thought, and bizarre thinking were all outside the range of anything normally expectable from the stresses of childbirth and mothering. Her family history of psychiatric illness and personal history of postpartum depression placed her at high risk for repeat postpartum depression. Her symptoms had not responded well to initial trials of antidepressant and antipsychotic medications. However, any beneficial effects of these medications could easily have been negated by the emotional stress of her fears, guilty ruminations, and isolation. There would have been concern from the beginning that medication treatment alone could not suffice as treatment for Andrea Yates's psychotic depression without concomitant reduction in the climates of fear, blame, and shame within her family and religious life. Her psychiatrist was aware of her symptoms of psychotic depression. However, he may not have appreciated fully the extent to which her illness was exacerbated by her religious life and family environment.

Answering these questions often requires more than a routine examination in an office setting. Collateral information about a patient's spontaneous, unstructured interactions with family members, church elders, or neighbors in community settings is often vital for assessment. Functional impairments are often more evident in daily life than in structured office or hospital examinations. In daily life, a well-functioning prefrontal cortex is needed to manage ambiguity and uncertainty, to make moment-to-moment shifts from one social context to another, to show discretion by checking emotional impulses, and to gauge how intensely to express feelings. Most major psychiatric disorders, whether mood, anxiety, psychotic, or dissociative, show these kinds of impairments in daily life settings. Access to such collateral information requires a therapeutic alliance that includes not only the patient but also his or her family or other close relationships. Andrea Yates's psychiatrist appeared to have had only limited access to such collateral sources of information.

In the end, distinguishing a psychiatric disorder from unusual or idiosyncratic religious behavior requires a clinical judgment that is based on the preponderance of evidence. Even when the gathering of evidence is conducted systematically and completely, there still can remain uncertainty as to the role of psychiatric illness in disturbing religious behaviors. Yet this distinction matters greatly for practical reasons. Diagnosis of a psychiatric disorder points toward symptoms best treated by evidence-based pharmacological or psychosocial interventions. Behaviors generated by normal sociobiological systems require different psychosocial interventions that appropriately target the sociobiological systems involved. Because both dysfunctional neurobiology and errant sociobiology are often involved together, as with Andrea Yates, both sets of interventions may need to be employed.

Setting a Treatment Frame That Addresses Religious Behaviors as Psychiatric Symptoms

Framing disturbing religious behavior as psychiatric illness fundamentally redefines the character of treatment and the therapeutic relationship. It changes how the patient and others may view the patient as a person. It conveys an implicit request that patient and family members defer to the professional expertise of the clinician and most so when psychiatric medications are recommended.

These negotiations around the meaning of religious behavior may bode well or poorly for the outcome of therapeutic intervention. A successful therapeutic intervention ought to alleviate shame or blame. However, an intervention risks demeaning the patient if the patient or family members have strong convictions that the behavior is divinely inspired. It then becomes a hurdle in establishing trust with a patient or family. Attending to these shifts in meaning and power are the priority of concern in discussions about psychiatric diagnosis. It helps to listen, understand, and acknowledge the patient's experience and beliefs and then to present one's diagnostic assessment as a perspective of medical science, but not the only perspective.

Ms. Williams, for example, was a 38-year-old woman with AIDS for whom psychiatric consultation had been requested because of worries about her depressed mood. She was apathetic, had a loss of appetite, and seemed disinterested in recovering from the pneumocystis pneumonia that precipitated her hospital admission. "Today I asked my doctor to let me die," she told me when I asked about her story. She talked about her guilt for contracting HIV from abusing drugs. She felt guilty that she likely had infected others through unprotected sex. In a drug rehabilitation program, she had converted to a Christian faith. However, she was now ruminating only on thoughts that she had thrown away her life and hurt others in the process. No signs of hope, purpose, or compassion from God inhabited her thoughts. She felt her death would be a just punishment for the wrongs she had committed.

My assessment took note of Ms. Williams's severely disturbed sleep, inability to feel any sense of pleasure, and waves of anxiety. Even if her fatigue and loss of appetite could be attributed to effects of her medical disease, this spectrum of mood-associated symptoms pointed to a severe major depressive disorder. "It sounds like you are feeling the weight of your responsibility as a person, for your own life and for other people whose lives you have touched," I said. "This can be a good thing. Feeling this kind of responsibility might represent the maturity you have gained as a person. My worry, though, is how severely depressed you are. I am concerned that the depression is disabling your brain in a way that you are not able to think, to reflect, and to make wise judgments. Right now I think you are quite ill with depression, so much so that you cannot separate moral guilt from the guilt depression puts into your thoughts." I explained my observations and rationale for this judgment. "Could we agree to treat the depression for a few days and then, when you are in a better state of mind, have a serious discussion about your life?" I invited Ms. Williams to step into a new social contract. In essence, I asked that she accept a sick role in which it would be her clinician's responsibility to administer treatment and hers to participate fully in it. When she was again healthy, she could relinquish this sick role (Mechanic, 1986).

Adopting an illness frame for treatment is most important when there are safety concerns, particularly so when there are risks for suicide, violence, or serious self-neglect. One can say, "I do realize that you see no light at the end of the tunnel and all you feel is despair, but I stand outside your situation. From where I stand, I can see possibilities that you may not be able to see. Can you trust what I am able to see?" Such statements encourage a patient to put on hold interpretations of mood symptoms as helplessness, hopelessness, and moral guilt.

There are clinical emergencies where social control, not treatment, is an ethically justified priority. Involuntarily committing a patient to psychiatric hospitalization because of a threat of suicide can be presented matter of factly: "I have an ethical and a legal responsibility to support your continuing to live. I know that you may disagree with me. However, I hope that someday you are in a different state of mind and can then appreciate the actions I am taking."

Setting an illness frame for treatment can be balanced by an earnest effort to conduct the treatment within the meanings and assumptions of the patient's life-world insofar that is possible. Arthur Kleinman's model for discerning a patient's explanatory model is a useful one to follow when symptoms have religious meanings (Kleinman, Eisenberg, & Good, 1978). Kleinman et al. (1978) suggest eight questions to be examined:

1. "What do you call your problem?"
2. "What causes your problem?"
3. "Why do you think it started when it did?"
4. "How does it work?"
5. "What is going on in your body?"
6. "What kind of treatment do you think would be the best for this problem?"
7. "How has this problem affected your life?"
8. "What frightens or concerns you most about this problem or treatment?"

These questions help a clinician to understand the patient's assumptive world and its beliefs, attitudes, and practices that determine whether the patient will engage in treatment and, if so, in what way.

When symptoms have religious meanings, additional questions are useful to ask that go further in locating where the Divine is positioned in relation to the problem:

1. "Do you pray about this problem? Can you share with me the words of your prayer?"
2. "Do you have a sense that God knows a purpose for your life? Do you sense that God has hopes for the outcome of this therapy?"
3. "Is it your sense that your doctors are working in accordance with, or in opposition to, God's plan for your life?"
4. "I know that you are working on this problem in different ways, and psychiatric treatment is only one of them. Help me understand where psychiatric treatment fits within the larger plan."

Additional questions can be helpful when spiritual practices are not God centered or when a patient relies upon a supportive religious community instead of personal beliefs or practices:

1. "Do you have spiritual practices that sustain and strengthen you through illness?"
2. "Do you have a religious or spiritual community that supports you? Are there others whom you wish to be present with you as you go through this illness?"

Such questions help attune the clinician to the structure of the patient's assumptive world. From a patient's responses, it can be clearer what the options are for tailoring treatment so that it best fits the patient's world. It is axiomatic that a treatment is most likely to be adhered to when it makes sense and has a purpose within the patient's framework of meaning. Mr. Wiener, for example, did believe that God was compassionate. He realized that God had forgiven others with sins far more egregious than his own. He also acknowledged that some meaningful purpose for his living must exist. With this much, Mr. Wiener could consent to treatment of his depression. I commented, "We hope that the depression can lift enough that you might be able to see more clearly what in your life is important. We will hope that you can hear God's voice more clearly free of depression."

Other questions can provide subsequent feedback whether the mission has been accomplished:

1. "Since we began treatment, do you feel yourself to be more, or less, the person you know yourself to be?"
2. "Since we began treatment, do you find that you are more, or less, the person you most desire to be?"
3. "Since we began treatment, do you more easily, or less easily, feel the presence of God?"

Current psychiatric practices have often focused most on symptom remission and reduction of drug side effects as treatment goals for psychopharmacological treatment. However, symptom remission does not assess the impact of treatment on the patient as a person. It does not assess whether treatment has rendered important relationships more, or less, satisfying. These can include one's relationship with a personal God. This separate inquiry must be conducted in addition to questions about mood, sleep, energy, and medication side effects.

Diagnosis of a psychiatric disorder opens opportunities for a long-term therapeutic relationship, and more so than clinical problems arising solely from sociobiological religious practices. Many psychiatric disorders are chronic illnesses with exacerbations and remissions over the course of a lifetime. The need for regular psychiatric treatment provides opportunities for ongoing dialogue about the role of religious life in providing resilience in the face of illness, which can include formal psychotherapy.

Avoiding Professional Hubris in Diagnostic Determinations

Distinguishing psychiatric illness from idiosyncratic, unconventional religious practices can be challenging. There are practical reasons for making professional humility a committed practice when making diagnostic pronouncements. Problems abound with the validity of our current psychiatric diagnostic system (Kleinman, 1988; Blazer, 2005; Horwitz & Wakefield, 2007). Our clinical diagnostic methods are far from perfect in distinguishing psychiatric disorders from normal syndromes of distress. These limitations on accuracy warrant caution.

However, there are more profound reasons for bracketing the understanding that psychiatric science can bring to bear on patients' lives. Although the neurosciences have made progress in elucidating brain circuits and processes of neural signaling through which psychiatric symptoms are expressed, they have not made clearer the links between symptoms and the meaning of lived experiences.

Science has little capacity for comprehending the private, subjective meanings with which patients imbue their everyday worlds. Subjective meanings, however, hold great sway in triggering or sustaining psychopathology. Different subjective meanings activate brain circuits differently and thereby produce different effects on the body as autonomic, endocrine, extrapyramidal, and immune systems are secondarily activated.

A competent mental health professional brings the voice of science into dialogues with a patient. The clinician's other task is to learn from the patient about his or her assumptive world and to bring it as well into the clinical dialogue. When the aim is to relieve suffering, a competent clinician sometimes gives science the backseat, not the driver's seat.

Safety Assessment

Approximately 90% of patients who commit suicide have a diagnosable psychiatric disorder, most often one of the mood disorders or substance abuse. The role of psychiatric illness in the genesis of violence is frequently a minor one, but it assumes greater importance in schizophrenia, mania, posttraumatic stress disorder, and personality disorders. Suicide, violence, self-neglect, and treatment refusal are each behaviors, not psychiatric disorders, but psychiatric disorders often play important roles in their genesis. When a psychiatric disorder plays an active role, its identification is important because it may have specific treatments that help neutralize its risk.

An active religious life is generally regarded as protective against violence toward self or others. A sense of ultimate purpose for one's life, a felt presence of one's God, communion with those in one's spiritual community, and hope anchored in personal spirituality all can stand protective against forces that propel suicide or violence. However, it is also the case that religious beliefs and practices, or religion-evoked emotional states, sometimes drive acts of suicide or violence. How religion can interact destructively with psychiatric illnesses differs for each group of psychiatric disorders.

10

Dark Nights and Exaltation
Religion Distorted by a Mood Disorder

MR. ROGERS, 62 YEARS OLD, ARRIVED AT OUR HOSPITAL EMERGENCY room with scratches and bruises after struggling with family members, who brought him against his will because of their concerns about his agitation, despair, weight loss, and threats of suicide. After admission to our psychiatry inpatient unit, he paced constantly and struggled to open the doors. He brooded and ruminated over the guilt he felt for falling short, as a husband, as a father, and as a Christian. He felt he deserved punishment and God's wrath.

Mr. Rogers was diagnosed with major depression with psychotic features, based on his current depressive symptoms, history of depression, and family history of depressive disorders. This diagnosis was validated by a quantified Hamilton Depression Scale score of 25, which was in the severe range (Hamilton, 1967).

Mr. Rogers did not want psychiatric treatment, but consented under duress after his family members refused to take him home. After 3 days of treatment with antipsychotic medication, Mr. Rogers was better able to converse about events in his daily life. After 15 days of treatment with antidepressant medication, his black mood, impaired sleep and appetite, and anxiety began to improve. By this time, he had told how he recently had become worried about his wife's health, his adult child who was having financial problems, and his performance in his profession. His global sense of failure and incompetence extended to his relationship with his God.

At discharge from the hospital, Mr. Rogers's symptoms were much improved. However, he was adamant that the antidepressant medication be discontinued. As a religious man, he believed he ought to deal with life's problems through spartan self-discipline and faith in God. In addition, he felt embarrassed that friends in his community might learn he was seeing a psychiatrist and taking medication. He came from a local community where a person seeking professional mental health services might be viewed disparagingly, and people were expected to deal with their emotional difficulties quietly with the support of family or pastor.

Mr. Rogers suffered from a recurrent major depressive disorder. Rather than shielding him from depression, his faithful religious life, including his lay leadership role in his church, appeared to have heightened his vulnerability. Interactions between his religious life and mood disorder were complex and multilayered, including factors that may have helped precipitate this relapse of depression, other factors shaping how he experienced its symptoms, and still others affecting his sense of personal identity. All these influenced his unwillingness to seek treatment.

His religious life may have contributed to the relapse via expectations he placed on himself in his roles as a husband and a father, his intense moral self-scrutiny, and the guilt this fostered. A religious perspective that regarded depression as a sign of weak faith or moral weakness, a view shared both by Mr. Rogers and others in his community, stigmatized the psychiatric treatment that he likely would need for the remainder of his life if future episodes of severe depression were to be averted.

Major Depressive Disorder

According to current *Diagnostic and Statistical Manual of Mental Disorders* (fourth edition, text revision [DSM-IV-TR]) criteria, major depressive disorder is diagnosed when a patient has had for most of the preceding 2 weeks at least five of nine symptoms: depressed mood (e.g., anguish, sadness, emptiness, tearfulness), anhedonia (diminished capacity for pleasure), significant weight loss or appetite change, insomnia or excessive sleepiness, agitation or psychomotor retardation, fatigue or loss of energy, feelings of worthlessness or guilt, difficulties concentrating, or recurrent thoughts of death or suicide (American Psychiatric Association, 2000). When the severity of depression is profound, thinking can become distorted to psychotic degrees. Patients can become delusional, with rigid, negativistic themes, including irrational guilt that one has committed so much badness that severe punishment is deserved.

Major depressive disorder reflects abnormal functioning in brain systems that regulate moods. Among these, the ventral sector of the anterior cingulate gyrus and the insula are instrumental for the perception of emotionally salient events and the generation of appropriate emotions in response to them. The nearby amygdala prompts emotions of alarm in response to threat, while the ventral striatum produces pleasurable emotions from rewards. The dorsal cingulate gyrus, the hippocampus, and the prefrontal cortex keep in check the intensity of these emotional responses. In patients like Mr. Rogers with severe and recurrent depressive episodes, four of these regions have been found to show atrophy or degeneration: the ventral anterior cingulate cortex, the prefrontal cortex, the hippocampus, and the ventral striatum. Moreover, functional brain-imaging studies have found the amygdala to be operating at an excessively high metabolic rate in depressed patients. The neurobiological profile of a patient with severe depression is thus that of a person whose brain systems for perceiving and appraising emotional stimuli, generating positive emotions, and regulating intensity of emotions are structurally damaged and functionally deficient and those for generating negative emotions are excessively active (Marek & Duman, 2002; Jacobs et al., 2006).

Although research has documented these structural brain abnormalities and autonomic nervous system, endocrine system, and immune system dysfunction in depressed patients, there is as yet no established use of laboratory studies for diagnosing depression in clinical practice. Rather, diagnoses can be reliably made from a patient's history by documenting the pattern, duration, and intensity of depressed mood and its associated symptoms, as with Mr. Rogers. Supplementing the commonly used DSM-IV-TR criteria with a quantitative depression assessment, such as the Hamilton Depression Scale, best discriminates patients likely to respond to antidepressant treatment. The latter step is an important one because psychological distress from physical pain, demoralization, or grief benefits little from antidepressant medications, even though such "normal suffering" also produces sleep, energy, and concentration disturbances of milder degree (Griffith & Gaby, 2005).

In a depressed state, the brain's readiness to process information related to potential loss, threat, or humiliation is heightened. Imagining a good future is rendered physiologically difficult. Difficulty experiencing desire or passion produces profound apathy. Patients find it difficult to feel a sense of personal worthiness or to experience concern for self, often leading to self-neglect. The emotional experience of depression can be more akin to physical pain than to normal sadness. When severe, a depressed patient can willingly seek death to end the suffering.

Religious Life Distorted by Depression

Clinical problems that arise when religion and depression interact include exacerbation of suffering, nonadherence to needed psychiatric treatment, self-neglect, and suicide. Religious beliefs and practices that evoke a sense of personal guilt can powerfully amplify guilty ruminations that otherwise characterize depression. Like the Ancient Mariner sailing windless seas, bearing a curse for his killing an albatross, depressed patients sometimes dwell endlessly upon their sins against God, wrongs committed against other people, and failures to fulfill expectations for their lives.

Mr. Vardaman was a 50-year-old man hospitalized for treatment of an autoimmune disease and its complications. His internist requested psychiatric consultation after Mr. Vardaman commented that "I don't know whether it is worth trying to live through all this," but then refused to take an antidepressant that the internist prescribed.

Mr. Vardaman's symptoms were severe: He slept poorly, had no appetite, and experienced no pleasure in any activity of his daily life. He despaired over events he heard about on the television news. He said no help was to be expected from God because "our time is not God's time," meaning that people should not expect God to deviate from his objectives to rescue us from the plights in which we find ourselves.

In a second interview and joined by his wife upon my request, Mr. Vardaman talked on and on, often rambling, about his frustration with his children, about the sorrow he witnessed in the world around him, about his childhood in foster care. Interspersing comments into his narrative, however, Mrs. Vardaman told a different story.

Mr. Vardaman had been diagnosed with bipolar disorder years earlier after successfully recovering from alcoholism. More often, his mood bordered on hypomania, with too much energy and little need for sleep or rest. He worked endlessly and tirelessly. Depression had been a less of a problem over the years. As a couple, they learned ways to keep his mood from becoming excessively elevated, by insisting that he get full nights of sleep while also avoiding excessive emotional stimulation, maintaining an active sexual life, and avoiding negative thinking. Lithium carbonate and carbamazepine had helped with the hypomania in the past, but he took no medication now. Mr. and Mrs. Vardaman were close as a couple and wept together during the interview.

My questions elicited a surprising inventory of ways they had successfully managed his mood problems in the past, ranging from avoiding exposure to television news about depressing world events to careful sleep hygiene. Part of their difficulty was that they had considered his current crisis as a mood problem related to his bipolar disorder. They had not been using their time-proven methods for mood regulation.

Mrs. Vardaman told how she avoided despair by "trusting God's hands." She described times when this faith had brought equanimity to her life. She believed her husband should stop expecting so much from himself. I commented to Mr. Vardaman that it was no surprise that trusting God came hard for him given the harsh circumstances of growing up in a foster home. I wondered how he had become able to trust his wife so deeply. If trusting God was so difficult for him, could he trust her faith in him?

The two spouses agreed to meet with me weekly as a couple. Mr. Vardaman would take an antidepressant medication, as his wife encouraged him to do, and we would work on ways that they as a couple could fight the depression, building on the methods they had used in the past. Over the next 8 weeks, Mr. Vardaman's religious life served a central role in their efforts. Since he prayed daily, both spouses thought of scripture verses that he could recite in prayer to "rebuke bad thoughts" that invited depression. He said he would ask God to help him "take one day at a time." He agreed to begin attending his church again. His symptoms began to remit by the second week of treatment and were in full remission by the eighth week.

Mrs. Vardaman's participation in her husband's treatment was critical for multiple reasons. As his spouse, she could help him move out of his depressive apathy that had led him to drop out of his social routines. As one who shared his religious faith, she could speak with greater authority than I about his need for psychiatric treatment in addition to his faith. Their use of prayer and recitation of scriptures differed little from the methods of cognitive psychotherapy for depression. However, it was conducted collaboratively and tailored to incorporate the ideas, practices, and worldview that constituted his religious thinking rather than professional language about cognitive distortions and catastrophic thinking.

Religious Life Distorted by Mania

Mania, in which a patient struggles to manage an amphetamine-like flood of energy and expansive thoughts, presents challenges different than those of depression. The exuberance of mania is typically confounded by loss of a capacity to self-appraise one's emotions or actions or to temper their intensity. Mania can be difficult to distinguish from normal enthusiasm or passionate commitment. It also can be difficult to distinguish from ecstatic, mystical religious experiences (Griffith & Griffith, 2002, pp. 245–257).

Unless mania is due to drug intoxication or a medical disorder, its occurrence indicates a psychiatric diagnosis of bipolar disorder, which most often is a chronic, relapsing disorder. Bipolar disorder is diagnosed when periods of elevated, expansive, or irritable mood, at least a week in duration, occur in addition to other periods of depression. Bipolar disorder is associated with grandiosity, decreased need for sleep, talkativeness, racing thoughts, distractibility, heightened goal-directed activity, and excessive involvement in pleasurable activities that have a high potential for harmful consequences (American Psychiatric Association, 2000). When these symptoms cause marked impairment of work, social, or relational functioning, or when psychotic symptoms occur, the disorder is termed "mania." "Hypomania" refers to less severe states. Bipolar I disorder is diagnosed when there are episodes of mania and bipolar II disorder when there is only hypomania. Unlike major depressive disorder, treatment of bipolar disorder requires mood-stabilizing medications, such as lithium carbonate, carbamazepine, or divalproex, though sometimes supplemented with antipsychotic medications or antidepressants. For a religious person, an important concern is whether religiousness facilitates or hinders adherence to medication regimens for preventing relapse.

Ms. White, for example, was a patient with multiple psychiatric hospitalizations for episodes of mania, depression, and suicide attempts. She had stopped taking her medications in the belief that she need only rely upon the Holy Spirit and inspiration from God for her health.

"God has called me to be a prophetess," she exclaimed. However, Ms. White made no mention of her sleepless nights, harassing telephone calls, and intrusive incursions into the lives of clinicians she knew, which together culminated in her being escorted to the hospital emergency room.

"That sounds like a heavy burden to bear," I commented. "How do you hold up under that much responsibility? Speaking for God is a very serious matter."

"Speaking for God is a joy. God gives me my joy. I am but a vessel for the Holy Spirit!"

"The Holy Spirit needs a fit and pure vessel," I responded. "Everyone I've talked to tells me that you don't sleep, you aren't paying attention to your diet, and you've stopped taking the medications that keep your moods stable."

"I don't need those things," Ms. White retorted.

"How can you tell whether it is the Holy Spirit or the bipolar disorder speaking if you take so little care of your self?" I asked.

"Well, that is why people at church are worrying about me," she eventually acknowledged.

"It is my responsibility as a doctor to tell you that you do need to take medication in order for your brain to be able to attune to what the Holy Spirit may be telling. That is my professional opinion," I said.

"I know that," Ms. White laughed. "You doctors always want me to take medicine."

"And I know you have some concerns about taking medication," I acknowledged.

"I see all these people on medications here who are zonked out. I don't want to be like that. I want to deal with it myself. I pray and I trust the Lord," she answered.

"Do you think God sometimes might work through doctors and medicine? What do you think about that?" I asked.

"I think you are trying to help me," she responded after a pause.

"It is my professional opinion that you do need to take the medicine," I again stated.

"Okay, I'll do it. I'll take the medicine," she said.

In talking with Ms. White, I was aware that she perceived no problems in her interactions with other people. She was equally noncritical in interpreting surges of emotions and thoughts that she considered to be divinely inspired. However, she was able to be aware that others in her church were disturbed by her behavior. To some extent, she was open to my argument that her religious mission was becoming distracted. Perhaps she could hear my bluntly stated concerns as coming sincerely from my worries for her well-being. She agreed to restart a regimen of mood-stabilizing medications.

Assessing Suicide Risk

Assessment of the role of religion in suicide risk is critical when a patient is depressed or manic. Approximately 70% of people who commit suicide also suffer from an active mood disorder. Suicide risk should be evaluated routinely whenever depression is identified. Suicide risk assessment consists of determining whether risk factors place a patient is a category of heightened risk for suicide and whether the patient already has thoughts about or a plan for suicide (Shea, 2002).

Religion often serves as a deterrent against suicide. Religious beliefs and practices that mobilize such existential states as hope, purpose, agency, and gratitude protect against profound demoralization that can propel suicide. Beliefs that suicide is sinful also can reduce suicide risk. The quality of relationship with a personal God can be protective for individuals who feel comforted by God's felt presence or who sense God's purpose in their living. Mindfulness practices of Buddhism can confer a capacity to live alongside pain rather than be reactive to it, diminishing drivenness toward suicide. Religious communities—churches, synagogues, mosques, temples—also can provide protective social networks that help their members prevail against personal suffering, thereby reducing risks of suicide.

However, religion sometimes motivates suicidal behavior in malignant ways. When patients suffer from depression or mania, at least five different pathways can move patients toward suicidal acts:

1. *"God is calling me home."* A patient can believe that the only refuge from suffering in this world is to join God in heaven. This motivation is most potent when one believes that God, in fact, has prepared a place and is beckoning. As described in Chapter 5, Mr. Miller was admitted to a psychiatric inpatient unit after being found on the ground in a grove of trees having nearly bled to death. Upon admission, he told the psychiatrist, "My only hope is God's glory and salvation." He believed that the only way to end his suffering would be to trust that God would take him into heaven if he were to die. Mr. Miller was discussed as someone exemplifying an anxious attachment style in Chapter 5. This sociobiological behavior was magnified to tragic disproportion by its interaction with the anguish of his depression.

2. *Death is but a portal to a better existence.* In "ecstatic suicide," death is viewed as a door to an idealized, nonmaterial, spiritual existence. By committing suicide as a group, the members of the Heaven's Gate cult hoped to leave their physical bodies to rejoin "the mother ship" behind Comet Hale-Bopp (Wikipedia, 2009).

3. *Self-execution is a just punishment for sin.* A depressed patient can conclude that death is a reasonable punishment for sins, failures, and shortcomings. The impact of the depression is upon the exaggerated severity and finality of self-judgment. Andrea Yates's killing of her children was an indirect suicide attempt. Yates expected to be executed for the killings and considered that to be a just punishment for her wickedness.

4. *Suicide is reasonable when one has been abandoned by God.* Ms. Hicks attempted suicide by swallowing rat poison, surviving only after days of hospitalization in a medical intensive care unit. A month earlier, her baby, who had been born prematurely, had died after surviving for only a week. She had prayed for the baby's survival but believed God had denied her prayer because of her drug abuse. She believed that God had turned away from her.

5. *God's mission requires the sacrifice of one's life.* Choosing to die in the service of God's mission is a constant theme in acts of suicide by religious terrorists, whether of Christian, Jewish, Muslim, Hindu, or other fundamentalist faiths.

Religion and depression can interact in complex ways to produce suicidal behavior. Mr. Smith, for example, was a 35-year-old man who became seriously suicidal during a long depressive episode. He attempted suicide by taking a drug overdose and then lying down on a subway train track, hoping to fall into a coma before a train ran over his body. Witnesses alerted subway personnel, who halted the trains until police and emergency personnel could rescue Mr. Smith and bring him to our hospital.

Mr. Smith had a prior diagnosis of bipolar disorder with multiple past episodes of depression. Mr. Smith was also gay. His father was a pastor in a church that taught that homosexuality was a sin against God. I asked Mr. Smith whether he was glad or sorry that he survived the suicide attempt. He regretted surviving: "I wouldn't live this life anymore. I wouldn't be hurting other people." I asked whom he was hurting. "My parents and my church," he said.

"You spoke only about your church and your parents. Do you also feel that God is disappointed in you?"

"Yes," he nodded, with tears welling in his eyes.

"Do you believe that those in your church, your parents, and God are all giving up on you?" I asked.

He nodded.

"Do you believe that you ought to be condemned?"

He nodded again.

"I notice that you responded more strongly to my question about God than to the one about your parents. Are you feeling God's judgment more strongly than theirs?"

"I don't know what to believe," he said. "I believe there is a God. I believe that he ought to condemn me."

I asked whether he would consider speaking with a chaplain while here in the hospital. "I would like to do that," he said.

He had already agreed to psychiatric hospitalization for his depressed mood. I summarized our conversation about his relationships with parents, church, and God. Because we would not be meeting again, I expressed my hope that he would continue this conversation with the chaplain and later with his psychotherapist. It appeared that his survival might well turn on how he resolved the conflict he felt in these relationships.

Psychotic thinking exaggerates the potency of any these pathways to suicide. The interaction of religion, psychotic thinking, and suicidal behavior is discussed in greater detail in the next chapter.

11

Worlds Confused
Religion Disorganized by Psychosis

MR. BILLINGS WAS A 24-YEAR-OLD MAN WITH SCHIZOPHRENIA who was brought to a hospital emergency room by his mother because of his auditory hallucinations. Two months earlier, he had told a friend that he was stopping his medications. A few days earlier, he had started going regularly to the local Baptist church. He became preoccupied with God's salvation. After listening to the sermons, he developed a conviction that his parents had strayed from the Lord and were in danger of going to hell. He began sleeping in his father's room to protect himself from the Devil. He told his parents, "God was talking to me. He called me to be a preacher."

In the emergency room, he was seen by a licensed professional counselor from the local community mental health center. Mr. Billings revealed to the counselor that he was hearing Satan's voice telling him to harm his parents. The counselor noted this in the medical chart and concluded that Mr. Billings was actively psychotic and potentially dangerous. There was no state psychiatric hospital bed available, however, so the emergency medicine physician let Mr. Billings return home with his mother, with instructions to come back the next morning to see whether a bed might then be available.

At home, Mr. Billings began hearing Satan's voice shouting. He paced, and his parents and sister could not calm him. He felt that Satan was inside him and that he himself was becoming Satan. As family members tried to mobilize help, Mr. Billings went to his father's gun cabinet, removed a 12-gauge automatic shotgun, and shot and killed his father and then his mother. He shot at his sister but missed as she fled the house. He then killed himself.

Religious Violence in Psychotic Mental Disorders

Religion-related violence associated with psychotic thinking is rare but often catastrophic. Mr. Billings had previous relapses of schizophrenia symptoms. He had reason to expect that this mental illness would render him unable to work, would impoverish his friendships, and would leave him dependent on his family as an adult child, all in addition to his suffering from disorganized and irrational thoughts. The interaction between his psychosis and religious faith took a fatal turn.

An association between violence and religious delusions is not uncommon. A disturbingly large percentage of violent inmates in American prisons have been found to have religious delusions, often believing that God or Satan directed their violence or communicated directly with them (Scarnati, Madry, Wise & Moore, 1991). Religious delusions have led to suicide or to such self-injurious behaviors as castration or enucleating one's eyes as a concrete, psychotic interpretation of the Biblical admonition "If thy eye offends you, pluck it out" (Blackner & Wong, 1963; Kushner, 1967; Field & Waldfogel, 1995; Griffith & Griffith, 2002, pp. 244–245).

Interactions between psychotic thinking and religion, of course, do not necessarily lead to harm. Moreover, some types of psychosis-like symptoms are experienced by people without mental disorders, and some psychotic experiences spur creativity and personal growth. Clinical challenges can be perplexing in distinguishing among these different pathways when a psychotic patient becomes religiously active.

Psychotic thinking can be loosely defined as an inability to distinguish accurately between those perceptions that are mostly, or entirely, a creation of one's inner thoughts and imagination and that those mostly reflect events in an outside, external world. By this broad definition, dreams are psychotic when the dreamer is so immersed in the experience that one loses mindfulness that it is only a dream. Political beliefs can be psychotic when unhinged from any factual evidence and sustained only by their telling and retelling within a closed ideological group, as with denials that the Holocaust occurred or conspiracy theories surrounding President Kennedy's assassination. Psychotic thinking can be hallucinatory, as when seeing, hearing, or touching people or physical objects when others present do not; delusional, as when holding a rigid belief at odds with accessible evidence to the contrary; or dissociative, as when perceptions of time, space, or self become distorted or there is a sense of leaving one's body. The distinction largely turns on whether the experience would also be witnessed by observers other than the perceiver. As psychiatric researchers Daphne Simeon and Jeffrey Abugel have noted, "If one person sees an angel hovering outside the window while no one else does, we think of them as either a religious visionary or, more likely, a person with schizophrenia. If 10 people see the angel, it may be a mass hallucination, and if everyone sees the angel, then we safely assume the angel is really there, whatever the explanation for her presence" (Simeon & Abugel, 2006, p. 17).

Forms of "Normal" Psychoticism in Religious Life

Distinguishing idiosyncratic or unusual, but normal, religious experiences from symptoms of a psychotic disorder can be challenging. It is also a question that has not been systematically addressed by psychiatric research. Isabel Clarke (2001) has pointed out that both psychosis and spirituality are human experiences that have been consistently ignored and undervalued in scientific discourse because they are so ineffable.

Distinctions between realities that are primarily imaginative and those properly regarded as objective events are often not clear-cut in normal human life. Observing this, psychoanalyst D. W. Winnicott coined the terms "transitional object" and "transitional space" to describe the realms of human experience halfway between the subjective and the objective (Winnicott, 1965). A child's teddy bear is a transitional object when it feels to the child (and only to the child) to be more than a cloth bear because holding it conveys the same feelings of emotional security as being touched by one's mother. Works of art, cultural artifacts, and religious rituals likewise all exist in transitional space to the extent that the emotional experience they convey extends beyond the words and physical materials in which they are constituted. The ritual experience of the Christian Eucharist occurs in transitional space. For the believer, the sacred meal is simultaneously bread and wine (objective) and the body and blood of Christ (subjective). Both are felt to be real in the same moment.

Similarly, anthropologists have referred to liminality as the region of human experience located between subjective and objective descriptions of reality and outside the purview of routinized daily life (Turner, 1969, 1982). Liminality was first described in the writings on rites of passage by the French anthropologist van Gennep (1909). As the end of the 19th century, van Gennep noted that rituals nearly always accompany transitions from one situation or stage of life to another, and he described rites of passage as those rituals accompanying change from one place, state, social position, or age to another. He found each rite of passage to be marked by three phases: (1) a first phase of separation in which the person detaches from the former place or situation, as when a young man in an initiation rite is taken by older men in the tribe into the bush; (2) a liminal phase in which the status of the person is ambiguous, during which the young initiate is subjected to ritual acts that can be either degrading, such as beating or cutting, or uplifting, such as being entrusted with secret language and knowledge; and then (3) a reaggregation phase in which the person performing the ritual reenters society as belonging to the new position and stage of life. In traditional societies, young people are taken into the bush with elders, who prepare them for secret rituals with liminal experiences. In American society, attending college often serves as a rite of passage for young people in which they engage in experiences that fit van Gennep's description of liminality: experimentation with disparate social or moral identities, use of drugs to achieve altered states of consciousness, and membership in cultish religious or political groups. Liminal experiences are often associated with hallucinations, trance states, or other dissociative phenomena.

Hypnotic processes with individuals or in groups can produce psychotic phenomena through suggestion. Hypnotists have been able to produce a variety of positive and negative hallucinations and dissociative phenomena through formal hypnotic inductions (Kroger, 1977; Erickson, 1980; Erickson & Erickson, 1980). Naturally occurring hypnotic suggestion has been proposed as an explanation for perceptual disturbances that are religious, such as hallucinated images or the presence of divine beings. In Galanter's (1999, pp. 63–64) research on the Divine Light religious cult, 90% of the members reported that during their conversion period they, to some degree, "saw something special that no one else could see" and 83% "heard something that no one else could hear." These findings were not associated with evidence that the Divine Light was recruiting mentally ill people but rather that the perceptual alterations were a product of the religious practices and group context.

Closer to the boundary between "normal" psychotic thought and mental illnesses are drug intoxications, kundalini awakenings, and spiritual emergence. Traditional native American societies have long used psilocybin from peyote cactus to achieve an altered state of consciousness during religious rituals. Numerous people have experimented with LSD or other hallucinogens in order to experience altered states. Such drugs appear to remove top-down regulation of sensory input to the brain so that a person experiences the world in a more direct, unfiltered manner. Meditative practices seek similar aims. Siegel (2007) explains the usefulness of mindfulness meditation as dissolving top-down influences within the workings of the nervous systems, enabling a person to experience direct, simple sensory awareness of the surrounding world to an unaccustomed degree.

Kundalini awakenings have been described during meditative practices as an entry into a higher level of consciousness, accompanied by surges of physical and emotional energy, detachment from one's self, depersonalization, and out-of-body experiences. In Buddhist metaphysics, the meditator seeks to open oneself to the experience and to glean wisdom and spiritual growth from it (Krishna, 1971). However, the resultant emotional arousal can become overwhelming, causing confusion, disorganized thought, bizarre perceptual experiences, and agitation.

Spiritual emergence was described by David Lukoff based on his personal experience of recovery from an episode of psychosis, during which he achieved life-changing personal growth and accrual of wisdom (Lukoff, 2007). Such psychoses have also been termed "spiritual emergencies" or "visionary spiritual experiences" (Grof & Grof, 1989; Lukoff, 2007). Psychiatrists from Carl Jung to Karl Menninger have noted that some individuals have passed through episodes of psychotic mental illnesses to new lives of creative endeavors and mental health that they had never before achieved (Chadwick, 2009). Anton Boisen, for example, became a minister and established the discipline of pastoral counseling after enduring a psychotic episode (Boisen, 1936/1962). These experiences of psychosis produced transformational changes in people's lives that led to personal growth or insights that revitalized their cultures (Lukoff, 2007). Many accounts of spiritual emergence appear to fit clinical descriptions of brief reactive psychoses or, in some cases, prolonged substance-induced psychoses, in which brain executive functions are relatively intact despite dramatic hallucinations, delusions, and dissociative or psychomotor symptoms. Manic-like mood states appear to be particularly common in experiences of spiritual emergence, with elation, flight of ideas, and an expansive sense of insight into the connectedness of all things (Claridge, 2001). When assisting a person through a psychotic experience of spiritual emergence, Lukoff and colleagues have recommended structured, low expressed emotion environments for the person, sometimes including low-dose antipsychotic medications, together with efforts to help the individual make meaning out of the experience through psychotherapy or expressive arts (Lukoff, 2007).

What these "normal" forms of psychotic thinking suggest is that a variety of interventions impacting brain physiology—drug intoxication, sensory deprivation, manipulation of brain attentional systems through hypnosis, controlled communications and relationships within closed ideological groups, or meditative kundalina awakenings—may each interfere with routinized top-down regulation of sensory information entering the nervous system. The brain is then exposed to novel sensory patterns that can be interpreted as an awakening to a new world. The difference between a psychiatric disorder and "normal" psychoticism may rest primarily with the intactness of prefrontal cortex circuitry for working memory, executive functions, and emotion regulation as it responds to these novel patterns. During mindfulness meditation, these prefrontal cognitive systems are presumably operating at optimal efficiency, even as they are flooded by freshly unedited sensory input. This abrupt juxtaposition of reflective thought with raw sensory experience can become a formula for creativity. In schizophrenia, bipolar disorder, and dissociative disorders, however, there are diminished capacities for reflection, dialogue, and interpersonal relatedness as a result of impaired prefrontal regulation of other brain systems. Disorganized thought, rather than creativity, is then the result when drugs, meditation, or other means remove top-down regulation of sensory input.

What has led to confusion throughout the history of religion is the difficulty distinguishing between psychotic thinking produced by nonordinary but normal processes of human consciousness and the psychotic thinking of mental illness from brain dysfunction. To a great extent, this confusion has arisen from assuming that hallucinations, delusions, or dissociative phenomena emerge from similar processes in normal individuals and those with mental illnesses. Further confusion derives from the simple fact that patients with severe psychiatric disorders also have normal religious experiences and spiritual insights, and their accounts of religious experiences can present an intermixture of the normal and the disordered. These problems notwithstanding, we are in a better position today than in the past to distinguish brain disorders from normal brains operating in exceptional ways. When potential harm to self or others is at stake, distinguishing between "normal" psychoticism and psychiatric illness is enormously important.

Distinguishing Psychotic Mental Illness from the Broad Spectrum of Religious Psychoticisms

Distinguishing mental illness from normal cognitive processes that activate psychotic phenomena is a clinical judgment that is made most accurately by weighing multiple dimensions of assessment. With varying degrees of reliability and validity, different dimensions of assessment can suggest that psychotic thinking best fits within the broad spectrum of normal religious experiences or else points to a psychiatric disorder that may need treatment as illness. These considerations include the following:

1. *Is there a specific cultural context for liminal experience?* Psychotic thought can be limited to culturally prescribed social contexts that produce liminality, outside of which the psychotic thinking dissipates. For example, Galanter (1999, p. 70) described an interview with Ed, a new inductee into the Unification Church, whose mentor had guided Ed to spend 2 full days in solitary prayer and fasting:

> On the second night, he finished his prayers and read from the Divine Principle while alone in his apartment. Suddenly, he felt he was in the presence of the Reverend Moon, and heard the minister speaking to him directly "as real as we're talking now. I didn't turn around but I knew that Reverend Moon was there. His presence was as real as any person I've sat with. He told me I was doing the right thing and should continue on my course, that I would find spiritual enlightenment." Ed could not fall asleep, and paced back and forth until after sunrise, when he broke his fast. He had never had an experience like this, nor was he suffering from any psychiatric disorder so far as I could tell.

2. *Is psychotic thinking circumscribed within the context of artistic creation?* Poets, novelists, artists, and musicians have commonly reported extrasensory experiences during artistic creation that were hallucinatory or trance-like or that operated with the autonomy of an external being. Watkins (1986, p. 98), for example, described the experience of novelist Alice Walker, who spent a year in the writing of *The Color Purple* "speaking with Celie and Shug and the other characters. She experienced them as 'trying to contact' her, 'to speak through her.' Indeed, they pressured her to move from the city to the country, expressed opinions about her work-life, and enjoyed a relation to her daughter. They offered other perspectives on situations than the ones Walker identified with."

3. *Do brain executive functions appear to be functioning normally in the usual settings of daily life?* Brain executive functions for prioritizing, making plans, initiating behaviors, motivating oneself, and monitoring one's goal-directed behaviors and emotional expressions are often impaired in schizophrenia and related psychotic disorders. In contrast, they are largely or fully intact during artistic creation or liminal experiences. In brief reactive psychoses, impaired executive functions quickly recover with alleviation of stressors. Executive functions are most manifest in everyday activities of life—interacting with

friends, attending school, pursuing a career, parenting children—where impairments can have a devastating impact on social relationships and work performance. Impaired executive functions account for most of the social dis- *NB* ability associated with schizophrenia.

4. *Does the emotional intensity with which a religious belief is held and the amount of time spent preoccupied with it contribute to, or impede, the person's ability to function effectively in personal relationships, work, and other aspects of daily life?* Membership in a religious cult or an isolated, cohesive religious group does not automatically mean that a person has a psychotic disorder. However, religious cults and mental illnesses can share certain behavioral territo- ✓ ries, which fosters confusion between them. For example, both religious cult members and religious but psychotic individuals can invest such importance in implausible, idiosyncratic beliefs that meaningful participation in normal society is rendered difficult. However, those with psychotic disorders usually *imp't* have pervasive social dysfunction such that they function poorly as well in the disciplined, ascetic life required by many cults or ideological groups.

5. *Do religious beliefs and practices produce personal growth and a deepening* *good* *of relationships with others, or have their effects stunted growth and isolated them* *qus.* *relationally?* The capacity of religious experiences to stimulate self-realization and relatedness with others is closely associated with normal developmental use of liminality and aesthetic creation in the context of intact executive functions. Examining the fruit of religious experience is a strong validity test for its authenticity and nonpsychopathological character.

6. *Do religious beliefs resemble delusional thought forms, unlike the unprovable but rational and coherent propositions of a systematic theology?* As Kingdon, Siddle, and Rathod (2001, p. 223) have noted:

Good ↓

> Spiritual beliefs may be clearly documented and consensus validation within an organizational context (e.g., the General Synod or the Vatican) provided. Psychotic beliefs may be "thought disordered" in form: internally inconsistent, idiosyncratic, and disordered in their expression with new words ("neologisms") and tenuously linked together ("derailed" or displaying "knight's move" thinking). They may also be markedly abnormal in content, using terms like God, the devil or archangels in conjunction with aliens, government agencies, etc. The individual may not have ever previously expressed spiritual interest or belief but the origination of their problems, often when under stress, precipitates these beliefs. The beliefs tend not to be recognized by spiritual leaders in their community or elsewhere, though the overlap may at times be significant.

Psychotic delusions usually fall into one of a limited number of categories (Kingdon et al., 2001; Wilson, 1998):

> ✦ Misidentification delusions: beliefs that one is a major religious figure or a prophet of God.
> ✦ Persecutory delusions—beliefs that one is targeted for harm by demons, jin, or the Devil.
> ✦ Grandiose delusions—beliefs centered on the coming of a messianic figure or an ideal age.
> ✦ Belittlement delusions—beliefs focused on convictions that one has committed unpardonable sins.

7. *Are there other associated symptoms of a psychotic disorder in addition to such "positive symptoms" as hallucinations, delusional thinking, or dissociative phenomena?* Schizophreniform psychoses, as chronic mental illnesses, typically include "negative symptoms" such as apathy, absence of motivation, and social withdrawal; thought disorganization such as loose associations or flight or ideas; and deficits in social relatedness with failures to attend to social cues or to match actions to appropriate social contexts. Absence of negative or cognitive symptoms is characteristic of "normal" religious psychoticisms.

8. *Are there are identifiable biological or psychosocial risk factors for occurrence of a psychotic disorder?* A family history of psychosis in first-degree relatives is a risk factor for psychosis. A history of closed head injury, birth complications, abuse of psychostimulant or hallucinogenic drugs, or temporal lobe epilepsy are among the medical factors that can heighten risk for schizophreniform psychoses. Recent sleep deprivation is a risk factor for mania. Social stressors or family conflict are common precipitants for specific psychotic episodes within the course of a chronic psychiatric disorder. Although not absolute indicators, such factors add to the probability of a psychiatric disorder.

9. *Does clinical evidence suggest a diagnosis of brief reactive psychosis?* In a brief reactive psychosis, extreme stress or sensory deprivation precipitates psychotic thought and behavior in individuals who otherwise have no history of mental illness. Recovery follows alleviation of the precipitating stressors. Such stressors can include social isolation within a cohesive religious or ideological group, physical environments with sensory deprivation, or induction of extreme pain or terror through torture. For example, Fred, a 19-year-old college student, was attending a religious youth convention in Washington, DC. He belonged to a charismatic church and had previously spoken in tongues. During the singing of hymns and praising God, Fred began speaking in tongues

and suddenly swooned, unconscious, to the floor, "slain in the spirit." Upon recovery, Fred acted strangely, ran about in a frenzy, touched one person after another in a confused manner, and talked unintelligently. Friends brought him to the emergency room, where he received an injection of an antipsychotic medication, ziprasidone. After sleeping, he awoke tired but thinking clearly and interacting normally. He did not remember the preceding events. He had no psychiatric history. Although glossolalia itself is not associated with psychiatric illness, the emotional intensity of the religious gathering appeared to have activated Fred's vulnerability for an acute psychotic episode.

Brief reactive psychoses are commonly described in third-world cultures but are seldom diagnosed in North America or Europe (Kleinman, 1988). They are characterized by florid hallucinations, delusions, sensory distortions, and out-of-body experiences, but are not preceded by deterioration of the personality as typically characterizes progression of schizophrenia in Western societies. When stressors end, a patient with a brief reactive psychosis typically recovers with a good prognosis for a normal future life.

10. *Has there been a history of a psychotic disorder with a pattern of relapses and remissions?* Major depressive disorder, bipolar disorder, and schizophrenia each typically show onsets in late adolescence or early adulthood, with subsequent relapses and remissions throughout adulthood. Fresh occurrence of psychotic religious symptoms in the context of a chronic disorder likely represents relapse of the disorder.

11. *Has there been a robust response to pharmacological treatment?* People with odd or disturbing behaviors in our society are often treated quickly with antipsychotic medications, whether clinically appropriate or not. When new concerns are raised about a patient's religious behaviors, information sometimes is available about past responses to psychopharmacological treatment. A dramatic cessation of psychotic religious symptoms over a course of psychopharmacological treatment suggests that the psychiatric disorder was a cause. Treatment response is not an absolute determinant, however. In particular, cessation of symptoms with a first or second dose of an antipsychotic medication means little diagnostically, in that initial sedative effects may nonspecifically alleviate symptoms from many different etiologies. For example, Fred's improvement following a single injection of ziprasidone in the prior example was inconclusive. Any method of sedation or a low sensory environment might have accomplished as much. In other cases, steady attenuation of hallucinations and delusions after several days of continuous treatment with antipsychotic medications would suggest more strongly that the underlying source of trouble is a schizophreniform psychosis or psychotic mood disorder.

Use of medication response to help delineate these distinctions was illustrated by Allen, a devoutly religious young man, who was periodically psychotic from bipolar disorder and mania through his early adult years. For a long interval after his diagnosis, he rejected psychiatric medications in order to seek a cure through prayer and faith healers. During this time, his psychiatrist and psychotherapist could do little more than strive to keep their relationship with Allen alive through expressions of concern and availability during crises. After ruptured relationships, disability, and failed efforts to find a cure, he slowly reconciled his faith with a regimen of mood-stabilizing medication, whose ameliorative effects on his symptoms he felt compelled to acknowledge.

Allen explained: "When Elijah fled into a cave in the wilderness to escape King Ahab, a great wind came, but God was not in the wind . . . then an earthquake came, but God was not in the earthquake . . . then a firestorm came, but God was not in the firestorm. Finally, Elijah heard a small, quiet voice say, 'Elijah, what are you doing here?' and it was God's voice. That is what Lithium does. It helps me hear the small, quiet voice of God, not the winds and earthquakes and firestorms of mania" (I Kings 19:11–15).

This statement, however, represented a slow, fitful evolution in Allen's attitudes about psychiatric medications. He struggled to find meaning in his symptoms and psychiatric treatment that would permit his religious beliefs and practices to stay intact. Observable effects of the medications on his mood and thought symptoms became a forceful argument for their use and his acceptance of his illness.

It can be difficult to assess the clinical significance of nonordinary or idiosyncratic perceptions, thought, and behaviors when they are intertwined with religious life. There is no litmus test for distinguishing mental illness from normal religious experiences that transcend usual boundaries of human experience. Arguments have been made that the two simply lie in different regions of a continuous spectrum, as with high blood pressure or developmental disabilities, where illness and normality are defined by arbitrary cutoff points (Chadwick, 2001; Claridge, 2001; House, 2001; Tobert, 2001). However, psychiatric genomics and functional brain imaging do hold promise for better identifying individuals whose structural abnormalities in neural circuits and neurotransmitter receptor systems impair their capabilities for thought and action versus those whose unusual religious thoughts and behaviors derive from sources other than primary brain dysfunction.

In practical terms, the decision to label idiosyncratic religious thoughts or behaviors as mental illness, rather than "unusual but normal," is a major intervention that impacts a patient's sense of self, the character of the clinician–

patient relationship, and choices to be considered when intervening clinically. The wisest course seems to be a systematic, multidimensional assessment, where diagnosis of a psychiatric disorder is based on the preponderance of evidence using lines of inquiry such as the prior questions.

Psychotic Thinking Can Add Risks of Harm When Interacting with Religion

Religion and psychotic thinking can interact destructively in multiple ways. Religious life can supply the content of psychotic thinking, as when a psychotic religious leader is inspired by cataclysmic images from the Book of Revelation to try to precipitate an eschatological age through violent acts, a paranoid company employee attacks co-workers he believes to be possessed by Satan, or a patient with schizophrenia hears God's hallucinated voice commanding him to attack his doctor.

Psychophysiologically, emotional arousal from religious beliefs, practices, or communal living can activate psychotic symptoms in vulnerable individuals. Behaviorally, a religious worldview can devalue the role of psychiatric treatment, framing symptoms of mental illnesses as problems to be addressed by faith, prayer, or rituals, leaving patients with psychotic illnesses vulnerable. Struggles with persistent symptoms can be experienced by self or others as evidence of weak faith or flawed character, which unnecessarily amplifies suffering. Cognitively, impaired judgment and critical thinking associated with the schizophreniform psychoses and mania can render a patient vulnerable to exploitation by charismatic religious leaders who, in reality, are predatory sociopaths.

Mr. Billings's story tragically illustrates some of the multiple pathways through which interactions between religion and psychotic thinking can result in violence. Numerous studies have found antipsychotic medications, albeit limited in their effects, to reduce substantially the risk of relapse for psychotic disorders. Mr. Billings from the start had a limited willingness to adhere to medication treatments for his symptoms. However, his religious life further influenced him to refuse them. He felt called by God to be a preacher. He believed he should trust God, not doctors, to solve his problems. These beliefs led him to replace his medications with faith. The intense emotional arousal evoked by the sermons, songs, conversations, and imagery in his church worship services likely played an exacerbating role in his decompensation. The intensity of his pastor's sermons about the "plan of salvation" may have been simply too stirring for Mr. Bohannon to hear without becoming disorganized.

By the end, he was experiencing sheer terror as he felt Satan coming upon him, then entering and consuming him.

Finally, psychotic disorders, such as schizophrenia, often have impairments in executive functions that render a person vulnerable to primitive losses of control of sexual or aggressive impulses. According to the account from Mr. Billings's sister, he was pacing in an agitated state and struggling with Satan, but in the end lost the struggle for control over his actions.

Clinical Strategies That Separate Psychotic Thinking from a Patient's Religious Experience

A careful, step-by-step inquiry into a psychotic patient's cognitive processes often can distinguish between use of personal spirituality to sustain hope, purpose, and connectedness with God and other people and psychotic processes that promote confusion, helplessness, despair, and paranoia. Tracking the ultimate effects of hallucinations, delusional beliefs, or dissociative symptoms on a patient's sense of self and relatedness with others serves as a useful strategy. A person struggling with psychotic thinking often is still able to participate in dialogue that helps realign religious experience toward safety and growth. Questions that externalize a mood of paranoia, or fearfulness coupled with uncertainty about whom to trust, can be specifically useful (White, 2007).

Ms. Liddle, for example, was an elderly woman who had begun refusing medications because she was afraid her doctors were trying to harm her. She was in the early stages of dementia and appeared to have paranoid delusions. Her internist asked for psychiatric consultation to determine whether she had the decision-making capacity to refuse medical treatment. In the interview, Ms. Liddle said that she refused the medications because an upsetting feeling would come over her. She then became afraid to trust her doctors.

"Where do you feel it?" I asked.

"Down there," she motioned toward her stomach.

"Is it like any feeling you've ever had before?" I asked.

"No," she responded.

"What does it feel like?" I asked.

"It's like a 'cheating feeling,'" she responded. This fearful feeling seemed to be felt deep within her viscera.

"This 'cheating feeling,'" I said. "Does it seem like it speaks the truth?"

"I think it's the Devil," she responded.

"How do you keep it from taking over?" I asked.

"I say a prayer," she responded.

"Do you mind if I ask you what words you pray?" I asked.

She nodded and whispered, "Lord, help this to be a better day in every way."

"Does God hear your prayer?" I asked. She nodded.

"What happens with the cheating feeling when you say this prayer?" I asked.

"It gets quieter," she said.

In our conversation, the cheating feeling now was externalized both from her sense of self and her relationship with God. I then felt comfortable asking whether she also felt that her doctors, and their medicines, might be aligned with God's purposes.

"Do you feel like your doctors are on the side of God or against God?" I asked.

"I think they are on God's side," she responded.

"Do you feel that God would want you to take medicine?" I asked.

"Yes," she responded.

"Do you ever pray for your doctors, that they might have wisdom?" I asked, guessing that, if not, she likely would be open to doing so. She nodded.

"Your prayers weaken that 'cheating feeling,'" I said. "There is a medication called risperidone that also may be able to weaken the 'cheating feeling.' I would like you to take this medication, but also for you to keep praying each day. Would you do that?"

She nodded. She was willing to take risperidone, an antipsychotic medication, along with the other medications for her medical problems. There appeared to be no need to challenge her rights to make her own health care decisions, as had been the original request of her doctors.

As another example, Mr. Phillips, 67 years old, was admitted after a suicide attempt by ibuprofen overdose. On hospital admission, he was severely ill with lactic acidosis, renal failure, pancreatitis, and respiratory failure but now was beginning to stabilize medically. Mr. Phillips was obviously psychotic. He spoke to his nurses about smelling the smoke of hell in his room, hearing the voices of God and his dead parents talking to him and telling him to be a good person, and both seeing and feeling the bites of hallucinated snakes. He believed that he was dying and feared that he was going to hell. He said he wanted to be in heaven with God, which prompted psychiatric consultation to assess whether he might still be suicidal.

"This sounds completely terrifying," I said to Mr. Phillips. "How did things get so bad?"

He said he had worked as a window washer. His parents and eight brothers and sisters had all died of cancer, and he was feeling lonely, missing his family deeply. He also felt mistrusted and betrayed by neighbors. He wanted to be with God.

Although I suspected that his description of all his family members dying from cancer was likely delusional, I realized that this was the reality of his experience at this moment. "You must feel very alone, having lost so many," I commented.

"You can't let yourself think about it," he said. He then added that his neighbors were making false accusations against him. Then he told how he had found his girlfriend with another man.

"That must have left you feeling very betrayed," I said. He nodded.

"Was this when you began feeling like life wasn't worth living?" I asked.

"I took some Motrin," he responded.

I asked how he had coped with the worst of times in the past. He named a church he still attended, and it, in fact, had recently provided him with some financial help. It was a charismatic church where he and others prayed in tongues. I asked about his experience of speaking in tongues. He said it brought a feeling of comfort and, with that, the snakes would leave him.

"Do you think God wants you to keep living?" I asked.

"I think He wants me to live, but I don't know why," he responded.

"Do you believe God might have a purpose for you to live, even if you don't understand it right now?" I asked.

"I believe He has a purpose," he responded.

"Would God want your mind healed so you could live safely on the earth without being so afflicted by visions of hell?"

"I think He would want that," he responded.

I stated my concerns that he had been feeling unbearably lonely and betrayed, so much so that it felt as though his mind was breaking. He had wanted to die. But he did believe God intended him to live, and his doctors wanted to support that. I recommended that he be psychiatrically hospitalized to begin the work of healing his mind from the injuries that it had sustained. He accepted this recommendation.

The reality of a patient's experience can be acknowledged, even if psychotic. When the evidence is strong that this experience is formed out of the distorted information processing of psychosis, it is compassionate to help separate the psychotic thinking from the personhood of the patient and to draw upon elements of the patient's religious life to help manage the fear, distrust, guilt, helplessness, and other aversive emotions that psychosis imposes.

To a great extent, a clinician lends to a psychotic patient one's own executive functions and capacity to regulate aversive emotions. One's intent is to conduct a calm, dispassionate conversation in which ambiguous, uncertain, and confusing circumstances can examined with curiosity and thoughtful reflection. The patient is helped to assert a path toward hope, purpose, and communion that feels both plausible and compelling.

Psychosis and the Risk of Suicide

Five pathways to suicide were listed in Chapter 10 as risks for depressed religious patients. Each of these pathways can be exacerbated in its intensity when delusional thinking or hallucinations are also involved. Co-occurrence of suicidal thoughts and psychotic thinking should always be regarded as a psychiatric emergency.

Mr. Lankton, whose case was presented in the Introduction, was a 62-year-old man on renal dialysis after his cancer treatment had produced kidney failure. Psychiatric consultation was sought after he was found bleeding with his dialysis catheter pulled out. His nurses were concerned that he might have pulled out the catheter deliberately, but Mr. Lankton had made no threat of suicide nor had he spoken about wishing to die. As is protocol in a teaching hospital, he was evaluated first by a medical student and then by a senior psychiatry resident. They found that Mr. Lankton had some mild impairment in concentration and memory, not unexpected given his kidney failure, but no other abnormalities on his mental status examination. He denied having suicidal thoughts or any symptoms of a mood, anxiety, or psychotic disorder. When I met him in my role as the faculty supervisor, I felt uneasy about the situation, in part because denials of suicidal ideation are notoriously unreliable when patients with a firm decision to die hide their intent from clinicians who might try to stop them (Busch, Fawcett, & Jacobs, 2003). I asked Mr. Lankton to tell me the story of his illness, seeking a detailed account of the events leading to his hospitalization and how he had experienced them. A half hour into the interview, I asked him what his greatest concerns were as he was facing the strain of a difficult and painful hospitalization.

"I worry about them," he said, motioning toward the hallway beyond his door.

"The nurses and doctors out there, you worry about them?" I responded.

"I worry they will bleed to death," he said.

His comment told me that he was projecting his fears onto others, quite possibly from psychotic processes that he had thus far kept hidden.

"Do you ever worry that could happen to you, that you could bleed to death?" I asked.

Mr. Lankton did not answer my question. Instead, he asked if we could hold hands and pray together. I told him we could pray together if he would lead the prayer. He began by praising God: "Our heavenly Father, we praise and honor you." Then he said, "Dear God, please help the doctors to understand that when you call someone to be with you in heaven, they need to stand aside."

When Mr. Lankton finished, I asked him if he wanted on this day to be with God in heaven. He nodded. It was then clear that he was seriously suicidal in his readiness to join God.

I told him that it was my wish that he be with God, whether in this life or after it. As his doctor, I could not know whether God wanted him to join him in heaven today. It was our wish to provide care for him while he was alive.

"Is it your sense that God wishes us to help you?" I asked him.

"Yes," he responded.

"It is my best judgment that the strain from this illness upon your body is making it difficult for your brain to think clearly. I would like you to take a medication that will make it easier for you to organize your thoughts, to concentrate, and to think clearly. Would you agree to that?"

Mr. Lankton nodded his assent. I continued, "It is our responsibility to help you during the time that you are on this earth. For that reason, we will ask one of the nurses to be here with you in your room to make sure that you stay safe from harm." With a nurse sitter for safety, a low dose of an antipsychotic medication, and continuing support from his family, who were alerted to his level of distress, Mr. Lankton completed his inpatient treatment and returned home without further psychotic thinking or suicidal thoughts.

Psychotic Disorders and Religious Violence

Psychotic thinking can at times propel violence toward other people. When intermixed with religious justifications for violence, the risks of lethality escalate as a result of dissolution of guilt or other inhibiting moral factors that are preempted by the religious rationale. This was evident with Andrea Yates, whose religious but psychotic reasoning overrode a mother's instinctive protection of her children. For Mr. Billings, religious delusions overrode a child's desire to protect his parents.

Mania carries special risks for religious violence in that it adds to psychotic thinking a high-energy state that is primed for action. Mania can contribute to the risk of violence through multiple routes. Like someone intoxicated with amphetamines, a manic patient is in a state of extreme arousal over which he or she has limited control. Its euphoria can give rise to grandiose thoughts about one's importance or mission in life or personal power. Self-appraisal is impaired and impulse control is low. When mania is intense, paranoid or grandiose thoughts become frankly delusional, and thoughts disorganize into auditory hallucinations.

It can be helpful to keep in mind a list of common pathways through which religion and psychotic thinking can intermix to produce violence (Shea, 2002):

+ Command hallucinations, in which God or other supernatural beings direct the psychotic individual to commit violence.
+ Grandiose or paranoid delusions, in which someone must be harmed or killed in order for higher purposes to be fulfilled, such as the ushering in of an ideal age of history.
+ Delusions of alien control, in which a person feels him- or herself to be possessed and under the control of Satan, demons, jin, or other supernatural forces.
+ Destructive entitlement, in which a psychotic individual believes that someone must be harmed in order for the cause of justice to be satisfied and personal woundedness healed.

Sometimes a hypomanic or manic patient can be empathically engaged in a manner that separates person from disorder, as in pointing out how heavy the burden is to carry responsibility for the fate of the world on one's shoulders. At other times, it is more effective to engage the patient's family in helping contain grandiose or impulsive behavior. Sometimes patients will agree to accept medication with some degree of coercion from family or friends, even though they see no need for it. David Kingdon and colleagues have described cognitive-behavioral psychotherapeutic strategies that help patients manage religious hallucinations or delusions (Kingdon & Turkingdon, 1991, 1994; Kingdon et al., 2001). Mills (2001) has proposed the usefulness of mindfulness exercises to help patients keep body arousal below the threshold of alarm that triggers paranoia and other psychotic processes.

Safety is a preeminent priority. When measures to collaborate with patients fail, it sometimes is necessary to state, "It is my best professional judgment that you are too ill right now to stay safe or to enable other people to be safe. I do know that you see this differently and disagree with my decision. However, it is my ethical and legal responsibility to insist that you be hospitalized."

12

Fear and Dread
Religion Shrunken by an Anxiety Disorder

IN 1678 JOHN BUNYAN, A LITTLE-SCHOOLED BAPTIST MINISTER in Elstow, England, published *Pilgrim's Progress*, a book that became the most widely read religious allegory in the English language. From the outside, Bunyan's life was noneventful. As a young man, he served in the army, followed his father into the tinker's trade, and married a young woman who he described as "amiable and religious." From the inside, his experience of this life was far different. By his recollections, his youth was recklessly immoral, lived with abandon as the "chief of sinners," daring God's vengeance (Bunyan, 1666/1987). Although his listed sins today might seem puzzlingly slight—profanity, dancing, and bell ringing—Bunyan was afflicted by an inner con-√ viction that he had committed unpardonable sins. Bunyan was filled with constant worries about the security of his salvation. His guilt besieged him. His felt experience was that of living amidst moral cataclysms. An inner voice spoke, "Wilt thou leave thy sins and go to heaven or have thy sins and go to hell?"

Bunyan began to preach publicly and became a thorn in the side of the official Anglican Church. The Puritan doctrines he preached resulted in two jail terms. During his time in prison, he conceived of *Pilgrim's Progress*, whose narrative displayed Bunyan's own moral torment.

Pilgrim's Progress is the tale of Christian, a man who seeks deliverance from a great burden that weighs upon him. Christian leaves his wife, children, and their hometown—the City of Destruction—to journey through the Wicket Gate toward the Celestial City, where he hopes to be delivered of his burden. En route to the Celestial City, he encounters Mr. Worldly Wiseman, who advises that he seek instead deliverance through the Law, with assistance from two other citizens, Mr. Legality and his son, Civility. Diverted from his journey, Christian, walks toward the home of Mr. Legality. Fortunately, however, he encounters Evangelist, who redirects him back toward the Celestial City via the straight and narrow King's Highway. There he meets Good Will, who points him forward toward the place of deliverance. Good Will at the end of the journey turns out to be Jesus Christ.

Were he to be evaluated in a psychiatrist's office in our time, John Bunyan likely would be diagnosed with obsessive–compulsive disorder (OCD), an anxiety disorder with a well-deserved reputation for the suffering it afflicts. This diagnosis would not mean that Bunyan's religious commitment, moral reflections, and acts of courage had no theological merits, but that his psychiatric disorder may have helped shape their form and intensity. *Pilgrim's Progress* implies that Christian's journey models a plan of salvation from life's burdens. However, Christian's journey, in fact, points out some of the ways that an anxiety disorder impoverishes religious life:

+ Christian abandoned his wife and children in order to pursue his own deliverance.
+ Over the course of the journey, no other person's life appears to have been particularly enriched by encountering Christian.
+ Christian's life seems absent of joy or exuberance.
+ Christian's journey produced no creative endeavors, productive work, or other activities that somehow might contribute to the world around him.

One can contrast Christian's life with that of St. Francis of Assisi, whose joyful celebration of God's creation has been legendary, or Mother Theresa, whose compassion lifted the suffering of those who were untouchable in India.

Anxiety disorders bring a surplus of needless suffering into people's lives. Anxiety produces fearfulness and self-absorption, which constricts relationships. Unlike a psychotic disorder, an anxiety disorder does not so much add idiosyncratic religious ideas or practices as impoverish important sectors of life. Although mood and psychotic disorders sometimes threaten violence, anxiety disorders rarely do. Anxiety disorders keep a person from feeling the joy and beauty of life, including that of religious life. Life's energy becomes dissipated in worry, dread, and bracing oneself for catastrophe.

Anxiety Disorders as Psychopathology

An anxiety disorder reflects a vulnerability to frequent or persistent discomfort as a result of:

+ Thoughts or images that evoke fear, apprehension, dread, shame, or humiliation.
+ Awareness of physiological sensations that accompany fear and vigilance.
+ Behavioral responses focused on survival and defense rather than creative endeavors or enjoyment of life.

Taken as a whole, anxiety disorders are the most prevalent psychiatric illnesses in the general population. They are important in part because they bear a high comorbidity for alcohol and drug abuse. Three anxiety disorders—posttraumatic stress disorder (PTSD), panic disorder, and generalized anxiety disorder—are major causes of medically unexplained physical symptoms in primary care settings. Untreated anxiety in a suicidal patient can be an ominous sign of suicide risk (Busch et al., 2003).

Neurobiologically, anxiety disorders occur because brain systems that alert to threat or insecurity activate too easily or fail to de-arouse after activation. To a great extent, the different anxiety disorders share a common pathophysiology. The amygdala with its threat-detection systems shows abnormally heightened metabolic activity. Brain systems that modulate the level of amygdala activation, such as the prefrontal cortex, dorsal cingulate gyrus, and hippocampus, are hypoactive. OCD is an outlier, in that it is associated with metabolic abnormalities in the basal ganglia, an area centrally involved in mammalian grooming and nesting behaviors.

Anxiety disorders appear to originate from different sources. Genetic factors, such as the homozygous variant for a short-arm allele of the serotonin transporter gene, place a person at high risk for an anxiety disorder if the person also encounters harsh circumstances, such as an abusive childhood. Early life emotional neglect or abuse has often been identified as a risk factor. Traumatic life events in childhood or adult life that produce intense and prolonged terror, horror, helplessness, or humiliation are also risk factors.

Accurate diagnosis of an anxiety disorder is important because typical coping strategies for the usual stresses of daily life are often ineffective in controlling its symptoms. In religious life, prayer, study of sacred scriptures, spiritual practices, and reliance on one's religious community for emotional support might partially buffer the severity of an anxiety disorder but typically fall short of controlling its symptoms. Unfortunately, intractable symptoms then may be interpreted by self or others as a sign of inadequate faith, poor spiritual discipline, or God's deserved punishment.

The Different Anxiety Disorders

There are different types of anxiety disorders. However, it is not yet clear from psychiatric research whether some may be simple variants of a common disorder, as are different colors of the same flower. This question awaits answers from genomics research and elucidation of involved brain circuitry for each of the disorders.

Generalized anxiety disorder is characterized by persistent worry about events of daily life combined with heightened physiological arousal. The duration, frequency, and intensity of anxiety are unreasonably intense for the level of threat. Common symptoms include restlessness or feeling keyed up, fatigue, difficulty concentrating, irritability, tense muscles, and poor sleep. Symptoms commonly appear in the mid-20s and are often lifelong (Papp & Kleber, 2002). In religious life, as in community life, generalized anxiety shifts attention away from plenitude and toward potential for catastrophe. Closely akin, social anxiety disorder shares most of the same symptoms of generalized anxiety disorder, but symptoms are mainly localized to contexts of social scrutiny, as when meeting a new acquaintance, making a public presentation, or entering a social gathering. Generalized anxiety disorder biases religious life toward fearfulness and dread.

Panic disorder is characterized by frequent panic attacks (Pollack et al., 2002). In a panic attack, there is a sudden onset of fear or a feeling of losing control, joined by such physical symptoms as hunger for air, palpitations, sweating, trembling, dizziness, and hot and cold flashes. Panic attacks can be associated with phobias, which is fearfulness about specific objects or situations. Agoraphobia, or fear of being trapped in a place from which escape might be difficult, frequently accompanies panic disorder (Pollack, Smoller, Otta, Scott, & Rosenbaum, 2002). Panic disorder and PTSD are associated with high rates of medical health care use because anxiety symptoms are misinterpreted as symptoms of physical disease. In religious life, panic disorder propels flight from perceived threats and a frantic search for security in God.

OCD is a chronic psychiatric disorder characterized by a range of obsessive thoughts and compulsive behaviors. Obsessions are recurrent or persistent thoughts, images, or impulses that a patient considers inappropriate but cannot control with willpower (e.g., aggressive or sexual thoughts, fears of contamination, pathological doubt). Compulsions are repetitive acts felt to have an irresistible urgency (e.g., cleaning, checking, counting) (Eisen & Rasmussen, 2002). OCD turns moral guilt into self-flagellation. It uses the energy of religious life to drive rituals intended to undo the badness of blasphemous thoughts or immoral impulses.

Patients with PTSD demonstrate chronic reexperiencing symptoms (nightmares, flashbacks), avoidance symptoms (emotional numbing, behavioral avoidance of reminders of trauma), and hyperarousal symptoms (insomnia, irritability, excessive startle reflex) after a traumatic life event. To count as traumatic, a stressful event must be severe enough to evoke terror, horror, helplessness, or humiliation that is both intense and prolonged (McFarlane, 2002). In PTSD, religious life can become dominated by its preoccupation with past traumatic events to the exclusion of other concerns.

Somatoform disorders can be added to a discussion of anxiety disorders, although they are given their own separate section in the current DSM-IV-TR psychiatric diagnostic system. A somatoform disorder is diagnosed when a symptom of neurological disease, such as paralysis, blindness, numbness, or loss of conscious awareness, can be shown to be caused by psychological factors rather than neurological disease. In religious life, somatoform disorders divert attention away from authentic moral conflicts because of their preoccupation with bodily symptoms.

Treatment of Anxiety Disorders

As with their pathophysiology, the different anxiety disorders share similar psychiatric therapeutics. For example, all anxiety disorders show symptom improvement when treated with selective serotonin reuptake inhibitor antidepressants. All anxiety disorders can be effectively treated with cognitive-behavioral psychotherapy that targets catastrophic thought patterns and helps the anxious person to desensitize fears. Some anxiety disorders, such as OCD, require more specific dosing of medications. Although many other antidepressant medications are effective as well for anxiety disorder treatment, not all that successfully treat depression will also treat panic disorder or OCD. Some anxiety disorders, such as PTSD and phobic anxiety, require specific psychotherapeutic or behavioral therapies and may be unresponsive to medications as the sole treatment (Davidson & Connor, 2004).

Most patients with an anxiety disorder need a treatment program, not simply medication. A full treatment program includes education about the disorder, medication, psychotherapy or behavioral therapy, interventions to optimize the quality of one's relational world, and incorporation of lifestyle changes such as aerobic exercise, yoga, meditation, and other approaches to stress management.

Clinical Problems in Religious Life from Anxiety Disorders

Regardless of the specific anxiety disorder, clinical problems emerge similarly when religious life is infiltrated by any of the anxiety disorders. Problems usually involve exaggerated personal suffering and unrealized possibilities for relationships. Anxiety disorders are strongly associated with anxious and avoidant-insecure attachment styles. A relationship with a personal God can become a source of apprehension, rather than a solace, because there is no confidence in its security. Interpersonal relationships tend to become organized by the anxious person's apprehension. The enjoyment of communing with others is lost.

Ms. Gates and Mr. Sanders: Happiness Stripped by OCD

Ms. Gates, for example, was a 42-year-old woman referred by her Christian Orthodox priest for psychotherapy. She was constantly preoccupied with a visceral sense of sinfulness as a sequela of sexual relationships during her early adult years. She feared developing cervical cancer as a punishment. She repeatedly sought counsel from her priest and God's forgiveness. Each night she could not fall asleep until she had prayed in proper order for each of her family members and relatives. If one prayer was out of order, she had to start again from the beginning. She felt similarly compelled to arrange her religious icons in a certain pattern and felt apprehensive if anything disturbed their arrangement. Ms. Gates was embarrassed about her anxieties and had revealed them only to her priest. Her priest referred her for psychotherapy when he found that none of his efforts to reassure her through counseling and theological reasoning were effective.

Ms. Gates gave generously to people all around her. She was the recipient of appreciation and affection from family and friends. Yet her capacity to realize her potential in a career or to feel happy in her life had been sharply limited by her obsessive–compulsive symptoms.

Ms. Gates did not wish to take medications for her symptoms. A lengthy psychotherapy brought to her awareness the sadness, anger, and emptiness that she felt in a marriage that was both childless and loveless. Her guilt and fears of punishment by God markedly exacerbated her obsessive thoughts and compulsive rituals. With eventual degrees of acceptance, she began refocusing her energy on future choices that might bring more happiness into her life. Her guilty obsessive thoughts became manageable even though they did not disappear from her life.

Like many who suffer from OCD, Ms. Gates had suffered silently for decades from her symptoms, too laden with shame to reveal them publicly. Because her symptoms were not so severe as to impact her functioning in her roles as wife, friend, and employee, no one would ever have suspected that she suffered from intrusive thoughts or compulsive rituals. Their presence was revealed only within the intimacy of a pastoral relationship and confession. The toll they exerted was not in terms of her functioning in life but in her capacity to feel joy in it.

If Ms. Gates represented the milder end of a clinical spectrum of OCD, then Mr. Sanders represented the severe end, where pharmacological treatment and behavioral therapies were obligatory for recovery. Mr. Sanders, 30 years old, was referred by his pastor, who had become exhausted by Mr. Sanders's persistent telephone calls and requests for counseling sessions. Mr. Sanders had come to doubt his salvation. Although he believed the Biblical scriptures ensuring forgiveness of his sins and his destiny for heaven, doubts crept into his mind. He feared he would die and go to hell. Meetings and prayers with his pastor brought short-lived relief, but doubts would return. They filled most of his thoughts each day.

Mr. Sanders had always lived a highly routinized lifestyle. Until this point, however, he had not been afflicted by notable mood or anxiety symptoms, nor had he sought psychiatric treatment previously. There were some strains in his marriage and dissatisfaction with his job. However, he enjoyed friendships and was a passionate poker player. His mood was only mildly depressed based on a quantified scaling of symptom severity.

With a diagnosis of OCD, Mr. Sanders's symptoms largely remitted following several weeks of high-dose antidepressant treatment. His anxious preoccupation with the salvation of his soul largely receded into the background of his life, with no changes one way or the other in his theological beliefs or religious practices.

Obsessive thoughts and compulsive behaviors, such as those manifest with Mr. Sanders, have long been recognized as problematic by spiritual leaders of religious faiths. In the Catholic Church, for example, Mr. Sanders's behaviors would likely have been addressed from a theological perspective as "scrupulosity." Scrupulosity is regarded as a type of sin in which a person does not place sufficient faith in God's promise of grace. From a psychiatric perspective, Mr. Sanders's religiousness had become largely co-opted by his anxiety disorder.

Mr. Madison: A Life in Flight Because of Generalized Anxiety Disorder

Mr. Madison was a middle-aged man who was hospitalized after suffering a ruptured vertebral disk from a fall, leaving him with foot drop and numbness in one leg. His neurosurgeon wanted to operate in a few days after the inflammation in his back subsided. In the meantime, his internist feared that Mr. Madison was experiencing an unnecessary amount of pain because of his anxiety. Since his teenage years, Mr. Madison had been a chronic worrier, tensely vigilant, and often sleeping poorly. He also experienced chronic headaches and pains and aches for which he regularly used over-the-counter analgesics and benzodiazepines prescribed by his internist. He would have been diagnosed with generalized anxiety disorder.

When we met at bedside, I told Mr. Madison that I understood he was suffering much pain. I asked him to show me the weakness in his leg muscles and location of the numbness. As I listened, I commented, "It sounds like you are scared about what might be happening inside your body."

"No," he said. "I pray to the Lord. He is my salvation." His tensed muscles *NB.* and vigilant gaze seemed to belie his words. I guessed that he, in fact, was frightened by what might be happening within him.

"I do understand that," I responded. "It is your faith that you rely upon to keep you strong. . . . But do you worry what these symptoms mean?"

"I am concerned that I've had my last chance. When I was younger, I used drugs. I've been infected with hepatitis C."

"Like your body has gone its limits—that this fall would be one thing too much for it to take?"

Mr. Madison nodded. He said that he prayed, and friends were praying for him as well. He attended church regularly and was trying to live a godly life. He wondered whether he was too far gone for redemption.

"If this were to get worse, how bad do you imagine that could become?"

"I don't imagine anything. I pray and God will care for me." I noted that he said this in denial of what he just spoken, that he feared he might be too far gone for God to rescue. I wondered what images might sit in the back of his mind, too frightening to look at directly.

"Have you ever known anyone with a back injury?"

He told how there was a man at his church who had no legs.

"Do you fear that, if your body has gone its limits, this could get worse and you could wind up like the man in your church?"

Mr. Madison whispered, "To say it in words makes it real."

I spoke gently: "Let me tell you how I'm understanding your situation, and you can let me know whether I have it right. You live a good life now—

You care for yourself, you pray, and you have maintained your sobriety. But you are afraid that your body went through a lot during the years of using drugs, and with the hepatitis C. . . . As you said, 'I've used up my chances.' In the back of your mind, you worry that this could keep getting worse until you are like the man in your church who has no legs. Does that sound right?'

He nodded. I then asked what exactly what was it that his doctors had told him. Had they explained the connection between the ruptured disk, his foot drop, and the numbness? Did he know whether surgery was recommended and, if so, what to expect in terms of recovery? He could not remember much of what his doctors had told him. It had seemed a blur.

I stressed my concern that fear from uncertainty was making his suffering from pain all the worse and suggested that he needed his doctor to slowly explain what had happened in his fall, why he had weakness and numbness, when surgery was planned, and what he could expect as a prognosis. Mr. Madison eventually concurred that he would feel better knowing what to expect. I recommended that he take additional medication to ensure that he would sleep restfully and stay free from the waves of anxiety that had been afflicting him.

In his religious coping, I was concerned that Mr. Madison viewed an acknowledgment of worries as an indicator for weak faith. This became an obstacle to his speaking about his worries in a manner that could facilitate communication with his clinicians.

Mr. Madison experienced an unnecessary burden of personal suffering. However, anxiety disorders also constrict and contort relationships in ways that place suffering upon other people. Ms. Finn, in Chapter 5, lived in lonely solitude late in her life because her anxiety-driven preoccupation over God's acceptance or rejection had helped drive away her children. They were bitter from her neglect. Although Ms. Finn's situation was discussed in Chapter 5 within the rubric of insecure attachment, she could also have been diagnosed with generalized anxiety disorder. Anxiety disorders are commonly associated with insecure attachment styles.

Ms. Brandon: Life Terrorized by Physical Panic

A 68-year-old woman began having episodes of abdominal pain that occurred suddenly with shortness of breath. She would become frantic and race to the hospital emergency room for urgent attention. Repeatedly, however, the emergency room physicians found nothing with their tests. She was referred to a gastroenterologist but his workup was also normal, other than some mild diverticulosis. Still she presented to the emergency room three to five times a week with the same symptoms. Eventually, the emergency room physicians told her that her visits were pointless and she should not return again.

Ms. Brandon was referred for psychiatric assessment as part of an evaluation for her medically unexplained pain. Detailed questions revealed a more complex story. Ms. Brandon had lost a brother and three close friends within her church, all of whom had died within 18 months of each other. She recognized that she would be losing more and more of her friends as she and they aged. Most significantly, her husband, 10 years her senior, was having health problems. She was afraid to leave him alone. Ms. Brandon's social life centered upon her local church, where a network of friends gave their emotional support. Her personal relationship to God, in contrast, was not one in which she could easily find refuge. Her inner image of God was that of "an old man" who looked down on her in judgment.

Closer examination revealed a symptom pattern broader than the abdominal spasms that produced her emergency room visits. She was frantic, as though she were lost. Physically, her heart raced and she felt short of breath. When her abdominal spasms began, she was terrified, feeling as though she might die. As these episodes became more frequent, she avoided leaving her home. For the first time, her husband had begun taking sole responsibility for their grocery shopping. She avoided attending church on Sundays. These paroxysms and associated avoidance behaviors pointed to a diagnosis of panic disorder.

Ms. Brandon's symptoms remitted promptly with a multipronged treatment program that addressed each level of her symptoms. An antidepressant raised the threshold for her panic anxiety so that panic attacks were less likely to occur. She agreed to a behavioral plan in which her husband would insist that she resume her shopping and church attendance despite her anxiety. After further discussion of her religious beliefs, she could state that the image of God as "the old man," whatever its origins, did not fit what she actually believed. During a psychotherapy session, she wrote on a notepad: "God is a loving God. He has to be the one giving me the strength and determination to face down the fear. That old man is not God." She carried these written sentences in her purse. She would read them when she felt fear building. The episodes of abdominal pain and her emergency room visits entirely ceased.

Evidence-based therapies for panic disorder focus equally on psychopharmacological treatment, either antidepressants or high-potency benzodiazepines, and cognitive-behavioral interventions that address catastrophic thinking, perceptions of entrapment or helplessness, and behavioral avoidance. Ms. Brandon's therapy employed both of these modalities, but did so within the structures and meanings of her marriage and religious life. She had long relied upon her church community of supportive relationships. The escalation of her symptoms before starting psychiatric treatment appeared largely related to the loss of these relationships as she had become increasingly homebound. Ms. Brandon's husband helped her to resume participation in her church community by helping her confront her fears about leaving home. She took on the cognitive task of restructuring her perceptions of God. Neither her formal religious beliefs nor her everyday religious practices changed over the course of her treatment.

Ms. Okema: An Unending Nightmare and Posttraumatic Stress Disorder

Ms. Okema was a 22-year-old refugee from central Africa. In her home country, she had been a daughter of her polygamous father's less favored second wife. Both she and her mother were often beaten by her father. When she was 15 years old, her father promised her in marriage to the leader of a neighboring village to whom her father owed political favors. The man already had three wives. She and her mother resisted her father's wishes for 3 years, but he finally gave an ultimatum. On a secret visit to the capital city, her mother helped her contact a humanitarian relief organization that helped her escape the country. Ms. Okema eventually was able to come to the United States, where she applied for political asylum through the aid of a humanitarian organization.

Although physically safe in the United States, she continued to fear that her father would pursue her. She began having nightmares of being forced to marry the village leader or face arrest by the police. She had intrusive memories of abuse by her father and was afraid to venture into public places. She slept poorly, began fasting, and lost weight. Then she began feeling as if her spirit was leaving her body. She had visions of being pursued by Satan but rescued by God. Satan would chase her to the edge of a cliff, but God would miraculously appear and rescue her. At this point, she was referred for psychiatric consultation.

In her initial interview, the severity of Ms. Okema's posttraumatic stress symptoms was evident. She was perceiving her father's face on strangers in shopping malls or public streets. She was having intrusive memories of being beaten with a rope by her father. Her dissociative visions of being pursued by Satan appeared unpredictably. When panicked, she had impulses to end her life lest she be forced to return to her family. She avoided falling sleep because of her nightmares. Her sleep was badly disrupted, her energy was low, and she had little capacity for feeling pleasure.

Ms. Okema was diagnosed with PTSD, major depression, and a dissociative disorder. In gauging her risk for suicide, the position of God within her nightmares and her visions was a key factor in my decision not to press her to be hospitalized. Although psychotic with her visions of seeing God and Satan and hearing their voices, God was always her protector, never a threat, and God consistently came to her rescue. Furthermore, her impulses to wish for death always came from her terror, never from God's bidding.

Ms. Okema was prescribed an antidepressant and low-dose antipsychotic medication, while also beginning sessions with a psychotherapist clinically experienced in African culture and skilled in the treatment of posttraumatic stress disorder. By the next week, her sleep was improved, her weeping had diminished, the suicidal impulses had stopped, and she had successfully managed her first court appearance in the legal process for seeking political asylum. However, she continued to experience some dissociative symptoms, feeling haunted by "a presence" that followed her wherever she went.

By 6 weeks most of her posttraumatic and depressive symptoms were in remission. Three to four nights a week, Ms. Okema would still have nightmares, usually about the elderly man to whom she had been promised coming to take her. One day she confronted "the presence" by shouting at it that she was a "a child of God" and as such held authority over it. The specter retreated and disappeared. Throughout her treatment, Ms. Okema continued to pray and worship in the traditional ways of a Catholic Christian. She prayed for her clinicians and for the soul of her father.

Ms. Okema's treatment had multiple components: efforts to create a climate of safety and security, education about the relationship of her symptoms to traumatic experience, trauma-focused psychotherapy, and psychopharmacological treatment for specific anxiety and psychotic symptoms. This professional treatment was carefully aligned with her religious faith and worldview that had supported her in escaping her father and seeking asylum in a strange land where she knew no one.

Ms. Jones: Guilt before God and a Somatoform Disorder

Psychiatric consultation had been requested for Ms. Jones, a 40-year-old homemaker, whose seizures were diagnosed as nonepileptic. Seizure-like episodes had been occurring during the previous 3 weeks. She would suddenly begin jerking in her arms and legs while falling to the ground unconscious. A neurological evaluation conclusively demonstrated that the episodes were psychologically determined and not due to seizure discharges in the brain.

Her initial psychiatric interview revealed the context of her symptoms. Tragically, she had discovered that her daughter had been sexually molested. The perpetrator's family, prominent in the rural small town, had successfully blocked prosecution of their family member through their political connections. Ms. Jones was pressured to let the matter drop. However, she began having dreams that she interpreted as a communication from God that she was responsible for taking action to protect other children in the community. She had not done so, and she began having seizures. Her physical illness was thus felt to be God's judgment upon her failure.

In a family meeting, the clinicians validated Ms. Jones's refusal to accept the community directive that she be silent. Supported by both her children, she made clear to her husband that she wanted him to take action, even though that might meet the ire of the community. He was visibly torn but eventually committed to act. Following the family session, her seizure symptoms diminished.

Although somatoform symptoms, as medically unexplained physical symptoms, are not classed with anxiety disorders in the current psychiatric nomenclature, they share with them the internalization of fear and terror. The triggering context for onset of symptoms has been referred to as an "unspeakable dilemma," in which a person feels trapped in an unbearable situation where existence of the dilemma cannot be safely revealed or discussed (Griffith & Griffith, 1994; Griffith et al., 1998). There was no role for psychiatric medications. Rather, treatment included full revelation of Ms. Jones's dilemma in a safe context, validating her efforts to protest rather than to submit, and mobilization of others to help her continue responding assertively. These therapeutic actions were aligned with her understanding of God's directive from her dream.

Understanding the Meaning of Anxiety Symptoms

Clean separation of symptoms into categories of either "normal suffering" or psychiatric illness makes for efficient clinical decision making. It, unfortunately, does not fit well enough in the real world. Grief from loss, demoralization from overwhelming circumstances, humiliation from stigma or injustice—each are different founts from which sorrows in their poignancy pour into people's lives. However excruciating, though, the sorrows usually go no further. They do not transmute into illness. They are borne and life moves on. When a concatenation of risk factors for a mood, anxiety, or psychotic disorder meets such sorrows, however, a new pathological process of neurobiological dysfunction can ensue. A new mood, anxiety, or psychotic disorder often takes on a life of its own, so much so that the original precipitating loss, shock, or humiliation is obscured.

In the prior illustrations, therapeutic interventions were conducted simultaneously at both levels, as the "normal" experience of suffering and as symptoms representing psychopathology. Intervening at the level of normal human experience meant understanding the meaning of Ms. Jones's symptoms within her worldview, values, and moral reasoning and then validating that meaning. Intervening at the level of psychopathology meant understanding her somatoform symptoms to be a product of excessive emotional arousal from her experience of threat and entrapment and her attempts to suppress, rather than to express, this alarm. A safe context was provided for expressing her alarm and organizing an assertive coping response. Interventions at both levels were conducted as well with each of the patients presented in this chapter.

IV

A Clinician's Stance

THE GAP BETWEEN THE DIFFERING WORLDS OF CLINICIANS
and religiously determined patients often seems unbridgeable. The
absence of a shared worldview easily spawns distrust, debate, and conflict. The stakes are particularly high when issues of violence, suicide,
self-neglect, or treatment refusal are in play. Concerns that religious
life is producing unecessary suffering are often raised. Whether or not
clinician and patient desire to interact, other family members, friends,
professionals, or governmental agencies often present valid concerns
for some kind of clinical intervention. What is a clinician's charge?
What can be reasonably expected?

A clinician meeting a religiously determined patient should
strive to find a position close enough for talk, but not so close as to
threaten. Neurobiological and sociobiological perspectives then can
help expand a clinician's repertoire, range, and sensitivity of responses
for opening dialogue, especially when conflict threatens. Establishing
person-to-person relatedness is a key aim. Categorizing, stereotyping,
and stigmatizing often then dissipate or fall into the background of
awareness. Clinicians and patients can feel secure in their vital identities and commitments while listening attentively to the other's reality. When dialogue cannot be achieved, sociobiological and neurobiological perspectives nevertheless can sharpen empathy, strengthen
compassion, and facilitate expressions of respect. From this dialogical
stance, "otherness" can prompt curiosity, not threat.

239

13

✦

Finding a Place to Stand
Conversing with Religiously Determined Patients

A HEALING ELIXIR OR A WITCHES' BREW? IS RELIGION MORE likely to heal or to do harm in a patient's illness? This book began with this question. By its ending, it is clearer that this question is not the critical one. Goodness or badness of religion is not the problem; religion obviously can be either in different situations for different people, in illness or health. The greater problem, rather, is how religious discourse can shut down personal reflection and silence dialogue, intrapersonally within the individual or interpersonally among people. When reflection and dialogue stop in clinical settings, differences between patients and clinicians become polarized. Polarization invites conflict, and discussion deteriorates into debate over which point of view will prevail. A solution for this problem is to reexpand the domain of reflection and dialogue, enabling patients and their clinicians to speak openly, to listen, and to consider together what is said. Sociobiology and neurobiology can provide tools for effecting this reexpansion of dialogue.

It might seem counterintuitive for sociobiology and neurobiology to weigh in on the side of change via dialogue with religious patients. Traditionally, sociobiology and neurobiology have been viewed as reductionisms that explain away meaningful content from religious life. However, sociobiology and neurobiology also can help structure interactions so that dialogue becomes more achievable, rather than less, and religious life becomes a richer resource for coping, resilience, and creativity.

The Problem of Mutually Totalizing Perspectives

Harmful uses of religion quickly put religious patients and their clinicians into conflict. The stories of harm presented in the pages of this text have illustrated repeatedly the challenges in sustaining meaningful dialogue when this happens. In Chapter 7, Ms. Bridges was in a stand-off with her internal medicine team, who were ready to force her to take antihypertensive medications against her will. Mr. Burns likewise was feuding with his neurologist over the cause of his symptoms. These patients' certainties were emanating from a religious worldview. Their clinicians' certainties were emanating from the worldview of medical science. Both patients and clinicians believed that their positions were truthful and correct. Debate and contestation characterized their interactions. In this struggle, each point of view sought to subsume the other.

Totalizing perspectives generate domination and coercion through the realities they construe. The gaze of a singular perspective redefines, reorders, and reassigns meaning to all that falls within its purview. Totalizing perspectives typically operate with little reflective awareness for how the act of perceiving helps form what is seen. They lack awareness of the emotional experience of the other, who may feel reduced, constricted, or rendered invisible by a scrutinizing gaze. As illustrated by Ms. Bridges's and Mr. Burns's stories, religion and medical science both can generate totalizing perspectives.

Conflict arises between religious patients and their clinicians when either party attempts to erase the perspective of the other. Differences can escalate into heated struggles. Sometimes the struggle for domination is not heated but cold, as in dismissive looks or tones of speaking or in simply regarding the other as inconsequential.

Sociobiology and Neurobiology Provide Keys for Unlocking Totalization

Totalizing perspectives appear spontaneously and effortlessly because they are anchored in the same sociobiological and neurobiological processes that have been discussed throughout this book. Attachment styles shape how personal narratives are constructed. Social hierarchy selects which stories of one's people are told and retold or are ignored. Social exchange guides which interactions in one's life teach moral lessons that are remembered in storied form. Neurobiology opens and closes shutters to the world—opening awareness of one person's pain, closing awareness of another, marking certain scenes or interactions as alarm buttons for entering survival mode. Individuals are pre-set to adopt totalizing perspectives as an initial step toward building groups that can be strong in their ingroup/outgroup boundaries and internal hierarchies. Neurobiological states associated with alarm or aggression speed shifts toward totalizing perspectives.

If sociobiology and neurobiology help build prisons of totalizing perspectives in which people become caught, then they also can provide keys for liberation. Few problems in clinical medicine are as baffling and exasperating as when patients act in ways that explicitly harm their own or others' lives, even though their actions are justified by religious beliefs or practices. The perspectives of sociobiology and neurobiology can help make such behaviors intelligible in a manner that gives guidance to clinical interventions. A clinician in conflict with a patient can use these conceptual frameworks to understand how religiously or ideologically driven patients think and feel. Accurately appraising the cognitive and emotional perspectives of a patient must precede any move to settle a conflict. This, of course, does not reduce religion to its sociobiological and neurobiological elements any more than art can be reduced to a chemistry of pigments. What sociobiology and neurobiology can do, however, is to give a fresh vantage point for understanding how religion sometimes takes destructive turns.

A Third Path: Relying on Sociobiologically and Neurobiologically Informed Perspective Taking When a Therapeutic Alliance Is Absent

Perspective taking informed by sociobiology and neurobiology provides an alternative to coercion when conditions do not permit dialogue or a therapeutic alliance. Well-trained mental health clinicians have broad repertoires of skills for relieving human suffering. These skills, however, were mostly honed out of training with patients who sought out professional help for their problems and, at the least, could collaborate in working toward aims that both clinician and patient could endorse. When a therapeutic alliance exists, patient and clinician jointly share agreement about overall goals for treatment, steps to reach those goals, and the necessity for dialogue built on trust and openness. Clinicians too often feel helpless when faced with patients who refuse such shared agreement. Religiously determined patients who erect ideological barriers can make clinicians feel as distrusted and disliked as members of some stigmatized outgroup.

One response to a person using religion destructively is to withdraw from the field of play. One can take a position that such a patient is not a candidate for clinical treatment in the first place. A clinician can affirm the patient's right to make choices according to religious beliefs, but refuse to treat unless the patient accedes to the clinician's terms for engagement. A second option is to suppress the patient's perspective. The right to make parenting decisions can be legally taken from a parent who refuses permission for a child to receive needed medications or blood transfusions, even if for religious reasons. A man who beats his wife into submission can be arrested regardless of what scripture verses he quotes to justify his behavior. A patient who seeks suicide as an avenue to join God in heaven can be involuntarily hospitalized. Each of these actions can be justified on moral and legal grounds when there appears to be no good alternative. When one has access to reins of power, extinguishing the decision making of those who disagree is always an option. Can there be an alternative to disengagement or domination?

Absent an alliance, a clinician sometimes is obligated to act unilaterally when interacting with a religiously determined patient. However, accurate appraisal of a patient's cognitive and emotional perspectives can enable clinical interventions to be conducted in consideration of the patient's autonomy to the greatest extent possible. This falls short of a mutual dialogue. Nevertheless, it does enable variable degrees of empathy and compassion. It can permit a clinician to act responsibly and ethically. It sometimes can even provide a platform upon which authentic dialogue can be built later. In Ryszard Kapuscinski's (2006, p. 73) words, "It is the will to become acquainted, the desire, the act of turning towards the Other, coming out to meet him, entering into conversation with him." This dialogical stance can constitute a third path between disengagement and domination. The clinical vignettes in Chapters 4 through 8 illustrate how this can be accomplished.

Similar issues arise when threatening religious behaviors are best regarded as symptoms of a psychiatric disorder. Psychiatrists have specific skills for treating major mental illnesses, particularly in the use of medications. Sociobiological and neurobiological perspectives of religious life can shed new light on difficult diagnostic distinctions between normal people who are acting in destructive ways and people acting destructively because they are psychiatrically ill. Only the latter are likely to benefit from psychiatric treatment.

Normal people acting destructively in their religious lives should not be regarded as psychiatrically ill. However, religion and bona fide psychiatric illnesses can be combustible when mixed, resulting in a disproportionate numbers of crises, some of which can be life threatening. Moreover, options for dialogue usually expand when psychiatric symptoms can be attenuated in their intensity. Accurate diagnosis of psychiatric illness expressed religiously is important.

Mr. Rogers with a mood disorder in Chapter 10, Mr. Phillips with a psychotic disorder in Chapter 11, and Mr. Sanders with an anxiety disorder in Chapter 12 each presented psychiatric symptoms that needed to be distinguished from the possible range of idiosyncratic but normal religious behaviors. Each case illustrated how control of psychiatric symptoms was a necessary first step before dialogue could be accomplished.

Emmanuel Levinas and the Other

The clinical quest through these chapters has been driven forward by evolutionary psychology and the emerging social neurosciences. However, its destination provides a fresh vantage point for examining more broadly the human encounters between clinicians and religiously determined patients. How do we better understand the meaning of these encounters? When considering our patients and their lives, to what do these clinical encounters speak?

Phenomenology, as a philosophical method, can help put flesh on the scientific skeleton that evolutionary psychology and social neuroscience have provided so that we can better grasp religious life in its fullness. Phenomenology analyzes subjective, first-person experiences of sensing the world. Phenomenologically, a patient who harms self or others in the name of religion appears as an alien presence to a clinician in a medical or psychotherapy practice or health care system. Such an Other comes as a strange and inexplicable being whose conduct defies normative expectations, either for how one behaves in a patient role or how one cares for self or others.

More than anyone in recent history, Emmanuel Levinas has made the ethical relation between self and others the most fundamental fact for understanding human existence (Levinas, 1961, 1981/1997). Levinas's insights help clarify how much is at stake in how clinicians relate to those whose religious lives raise clinical concerns.

Emmanuel Levinas was a Jewish philosopher whose response to the Holocaust was to make ethical responsibility for the Other foundational in understanding what it means to attain selfhood as a human being. As a French soldier, Levinas did forced labor as a prisoner of war during World War II, while his wife and daughter hid in a French monastery. His Lithuanian family died in the Holocaust. The reality of the Holocaust and the dehumanizing

246 A CLINICIAN'S STANCE

Nazi gaze defined for Levinas his life work. Emerging from the war, he devoted himself to understanding how systems of thought help make the possibility of war rational.

Levinas found the source code for genocide in an unlikely place. He tracked the simplest of distinctions—that between "same" and "other"—as this cognitive act had been dealt with by major bodies of European thought over the course of history. In the preface to his major work, *Totality and Infinity*, Levinas wrote (1961, p. 21):

> Violence does not consist so much in injuring and annihilating persons as in interrupting their continuity, making them play roles in which they no longer recognize themselves, making them betray not only commitments but their own substance, making them carry out actions that will destroy every possibility for action. Not only modern war but every war employs arms that turn against those who wield them. It establishes an order from which no one can keep his distance; nothing henceforth is exterior.

Levinas noted that the great systems of thought from the three H's of German philosophy—Hegel, Husserl, and Heidegger—were each totalizing in their fitting every aspect of human life into their overarching frameworks of ideas. Levinas proposed that totalization is valued because it seeks in "sameness" a refuge against anxiety evoked by perceiving the infinite. A commitment to the Other—the stranger, the outsider, the person whose experience is inexplicable within one's own worldview—opens up awareness of the infinite.

Levinas identified totalization as the bedrock upon which violence and war rested. Through his tracking of concrete patterns of everyday human experiences, Levinas argued that totalization is always fraudulent. He showed how every human encounter has multiple centers of reasoning among the persons involved in it. No single overcompassing system of thought can subsume fully every point of view. The multiple perspectives in a human encounter do not make up the pieces of a puzzle that together fit into a whole. Taken together, rather, they generate not totality but infinity.

Before Levinas, philosophers felt confident about the existence of the conscious self. As Descartes put it, "I think, therefore I am." Proving existence of other beings was more of a challenge. Still harder was proof that a fundamental ethical obligation existed from self toward others, which seemed to require jumps in logic, rhetorical devices, or divine revelation to make it stick. Levinas's analysis turned all this on its head. Like a chemist studying an unknown crystal, Levinas stripped away the layers of human existence down to its constituent atoms. Just as protons and electrons must stand in a specific relation in order to retain elemental identity as an atom, Levinas found a relation, not isolated particles, at the heart of human existence. For Levinas, existence stripped bare has at its core an irreducible relation between self and other—an ethical commitment to care and protection. Existence of a self rests upon an ethical relatedness with others.

Sociobiology, akin to Levinas, finds that the human nervous system has a space built into it for the Other. The human brain is mostly a social brain. Developmentally, the mirror neuron system and systems for appraising cognitive and emotional perspectives of others are already maturing, even before a growing baby becomes consciously aware or shows agency as a self. A space for the Other is already under construction. The empirical sciences of sociobiology and neurobiology, of course, do not speak from the same world as does philosophy. However, the science points to a human world that lies beyond itself, much as the architecture of our buildings gives hints of lives that can be expected to unfold within them. Levinas can help us grasp the core meaning of that unfolding world.

Levinas's concerns were practical ones. What can be an antidote for totalization if that is what sets the stage for domination, exploitation, and extermination of those who are Other? For Levinas the answer is a commitment to dialogue with the Other whenever it can happen, to whatever extent it can happen.[1] Dialogue supports a relation between self and Other, while still accepting and protecting the strangeness and autonomy of the Other. Dialogue enables people to be in relationships that are not defined by dependence or control. Avoiding either capitulating to or dominating the perspective of the other necessitates dialogue. For a clinician, this means building conditions for dialogue where dialogue does not already exist. When this proves impossible, a clinician still must go as far as possible in protecting the otherness of his or her patient by interacting respectfully and ethically, as if awaiting the possibility for dialogue.

Stigma is an arrow that points to otherness. Generally, any kind of stigma—moral, contagion, ethnic, racial, socioeconomic, religious—identifies people most likely to be experienced as strange, "not of my world," disturbing not only in their behavior but in their being. Religious stigma reveals itself in

---

[1] Here Levinas laid out a middle path between Jean Paul Sartre, who viewed all human relationships as destined to endless struggles to dominate each other, and Martin Buber, who sought mutual dialogue in I–Thou relationships where persons would be fully attentive to one another in emotions of reverence, acceptance, and concern. Levinas accepted the nonmutual, asymmetrical character of self–other relationships without relinquishing a commitment to dialogue.

countertransferential urges to feel disdain, to express contempt, to avoid contact with religious people when their religiousness interferes with their own or others' health. Levinas's directive is to put added energy into dialogue with such people and to protect their otherness as a conservationist would protect an endangered species.

Finding a Position That Favors Dialogue

Finding dialogue with a religiously determined patient can be like finding water in the desert: The art of success is picking the best place to search for it. Patients who present clinical problems arising from religious sociobiology rarely seek the assistance of mental health professionals voluntarily. Clinical encounters more often are forced through some degree of coercion by family, physician, school system, the court, or some other monitoring presence. Despite such adverse conditions, a clinician is asked to intervene, often in a single encounter or handful of sessions. The art of dialogue is finding a position from which it is more likely, rather than less likely, to occur.

Understanding religious sociobiology can help a clinician to find a position from which defensive sociobiological behaviors are at least risk for activation, which can tilt a conversation toward dialogue rather than debate. Awareness of religious group boundaries, roles and hierarchy, identity flags, and ingroup/outgroup kin recognition processes can help a clinician anticipate what may be perceived as a threat or simply "too different." This mindfulness is most important when the patient or members of the patient's religious group already distrust or feel contemptuous toward mental health clinicians.

Understanding religious sociobiology helps sharpen distinctions between sociobiological religiousness and personal spirituality, both of which may contribute to a patient's religious life. Whenever sociobiological religion dominates religious life to the exclusion of personal spirituality, there is some level of risk for harm to individuals within or outside the religious group. Those within the group may stand at internal risk for coercion, exploitation, or other forms of abuse or neglect, whereas those outside group may be at external risk for stigmatization, discrimination, exploitation, and violence. Promoting influences of personal spirituality expands possibilities for dialogue. Rebalancing the relative influences of sociobiological religion and personal spirituality can attenuate or prevent destructive uses of religion. Finding a position from which to initiate conversation is key. It must be close enough to make contact but not so close as to threaten.

The Seduction of Sameness

"Why put up with the nonsense?" can be the honest, if unspoken, response by many clinicians when encountering a patient who, for religious reasons, resists or refuses treatment, bears unnecessary suffering, or poses a threat to self or others. Encountering patients like Mr. Chin in the Introduction, Mr. Burns or Ms. Bridges in Chapter 7, and Ms. Bass in Chapter 8 is maddening for hospital physicians attempting to get the day's work done. The routines of medical care—treatment pathways, clinical algorhithms, manualized psychotherapies, evidence-based therapeutics—are designed to flow smoothly and efficiently. Religiously determined patients slow things down or sometimes bring treatment to a stop.

In his poem "Mending Fences," Robert Frost's (1915) neighbor tells him, "Good fences make good neighbors," as they rebuild the stone wall along their property line each spring. Frost views this work as pointless. He has no use for fences that separate people. He knows that his apple trees will not steal the cones of his neighbor's pine trees. However, a fence is what his neighbor wants. They are able to have a conversation because Frost heeds his neighbor's expectations and labors with him to build the wall. Albeit grudgingly, Frost learned where he needed to stand if they were to talk. Accepting the other as different from the sameness of oneself is a difficult lesson to learn.

A Religiously Determined Patient Needs the Clinician as Other

A religiously determined patient needs a clinician's persistent standing in his or her religious world in order to learn that no ideology, whether Christian, Muslim, Jewish, Hindu, or Buddhist, is sufficient to describe a person. This is true even when a patient demands to be regarded only in terms of religious identity. The clinician's presence stands in the way of the patient's faith. This standing firm conveys a message that relationships and dialogue are important. Expressing care, concern, and respect are important. That everyone should hold the same worldview is less important. The labor required for building fences is even less important.

As Emmanuel Levinas observed (1961, p. 73), "The absolutely foreign can instruct us. And it is only man who can be absolutely foreign to me— refractory to every typology, to every genus, to every characterology, to every classification—and consequently the term of a 'knowledge' finally penetrating beyond the object. The strangeness of the Other, his very freedom! Free beings alone can be strangers to one another." The worldview of cohesive religious or ideological groups seeks sameness and avoids difference. As a stranger, I bring difference. If we stand close enough to talk but apart enough so as not to intimidate, then strangeness can become instructive.

Clinicians and Clinical Systems Need the Otherness of Religiously Determined Patients

Encountering a religiously determined patient forces me, as a clinician, to practice, for lack of any better word, neighborliness. I find myself obligated to make space for the other regardless of my beliefs or practices. Like Robert Frost's narrator, I help build the wall my neighbor wants built because I want a good neighbor more than I want my point of view to dominate.

My hospital also needs my religiously determined patient. As corporate entities, hospitals value "through-put" more than nearly any other performance measure.

Through-put is a number that quantifies how quickly patients traverse the clinical system: in the front door, treated, then out the back door. Efficiency of through-put helps determine how much Medicare and commercial insurers reimburse hospitals and clinicians for their services. Optimal through-put means maximally efficient use of health care resources. Standardization of treatment protocols by treatment algorhithms and best practices improves the efficiency needed for optimal through-put. Through-put is about populations of patients, not any patient's particular life.

It can be propitious when a religiously determined patient stops this commoditization of health care dead in its tracks by refusing, on religious grounds, to participate. A religiously determined person sends the message "How you know me as a person matters." The appearance of a religiously determined person in a clinical setting becomes a reminder that person-to-person relatedness is not a natural by-product of the policies, procedures, and social structures of our clinical systems.

A religiously determined patient within an integrated, efficient health care system has much the same status as an endangered animal species threatened by urban sprawl or a local ethnic community threatened by an increasingly globalized world. Commitment to a protected existence for grizzly bears in Alaska or Bedouins on the Arabian Peninsula conflicts with the totalization of capitalistic free markets and globalized communications. Yet their successful protection is our own insurance that we too will be regarded as persons in our health care system, not as commodities.

Accepting a Role as Other

It is my desire to stay in dialogue with my religiously determined patient until "religiously determined" fades from the foreground, and my patient is simply a person. A person is not a person if known only as a category. My religiously determined patient may not grant that option, though, and it is then that I encounter my patient's otherness.

The theme of this book has been commitment to dialogue despite the frequent asymmetry and nonmutuality of interactions with religiously determined patients. This is a difficult stance because it denies the impulse to attack the strangeness of the Other. My task has been neither to make a religiously determined patient a citizen of my world nor to become a citizen of my patient's realm, but rather to stay in relation at a respectful distance, to "let live," with conversation, not coercion, providing our connection.

In the stories of this text, the religiously determined patients whom I have encountered have often needed me, as a clinician, as an Other. At my best, I have embraced this role, not one to dictate but to stay present with a different voice. I cannot fathom why the vocation of a particular person is to stand as representative and defender of a particular religion or ideology. As Heidegger poignantly put it, a person's being is set in motion like a thrown stone that becomes conscious in midflight, long before there exists even a modicum of self-awareness for grasping the meaning of it all (Barrett, 1958, pp. 219–220). We are all caught in our thrown-ness, discovering who we already have become, my own life no less so than my patient's life, so I accept this. For this process of discovery to advance, encounters with Others need to happen. From a position as Other, a clinician can ask questions that might never be addressed to a patient from within his or her world. These questions can be asked with authenticity, concern, and respect, but their unique value lies in their otherness. This view is a long-range one. The task is not to change the patient but to stage a dialogue. Such encounters carry the hope that a patient will become a more capable moral agent in his or her own religious life. Such encounters help my own humanity as a clinician to stay alive.

References

Abbott, A. (2001). Into the mind of a killer. *Nature, 410,* 296–298.

Abbott, A. (2007). Abnormal neuroscience: Scanning psychopaths. *Nature, 450,* 942–944.

Albanese, M.-C., Duerden, E. G., Rainville, P., & Duncan, G. H. (2007). Memory traces of pain in the human cortex. *Journal of Neuroscience, 27,* 4612–4620.

Albaugh, B. J., & Anderson, P. O. (1974). Peyote in the treatment of alcoholism among American Indians. *American Journal of Psychiatry, 131,* 1247–1250.

Alexander, R. D. (1987). *The biology of moral systems.* Hawthorne, NY: Aldine de Gruyter.

American Psychiatric Association. (2000). *Diagnostic and statistical manual of mental disorders* (4th ed., text rev.). Washington, DC: Author.

Anderson, H. (1997). *Conversation, language, and possibilities.* New York: Basic Books.

Armstrong, K. (1993). *A history of God.* New York: Ballantine Books.

Armstrong, K. (2004). *The spiral staircase: My climb out of darkness.* New York: Anchor Books.

Association of American Medical Colleges. (1999). *Report III: Contemporary issues in medicine: Communication in medicine.* Washington, DC: Author.

Associated Press. (2006, July 26). *Jury: Yates not guilty by reason of insanity.* Retrieved January 25, 2010, from *www.msnbc.com./id/140247281.*

Barabasz, A. F., & Barabasz, M. (2008). Hypnosis and the brain. In M. R. Nash & A. J. Barnier (Eds.), *The Oxford handbook of hypnosis* (pp. 337–364). New York: Oxford University Press.

Barinaga, M. (1996). Social status sculpts activity of crayfish neurons. *Science, 271,* 290–291.

Barnes, M. H. B. (2000). *Stages of thought: The co-evolution of religious thought and science.* New York: Oxford University Press.

Barnes, M. H. B. (2003). *In the presence of mystery: An introduction to the story of human religiousness.* Mystic, CT: Twenty-Third Publications.

Barnier, A. J., & Nash, M. R. (2008). Introduction: A roadmap for explanation, a working definition. In M. R. Nash & A. J. Barnier (Eds.), *The Oxford handbook of hypnosis: Theory, research and practice* (pp. 1–20). New York: Oxford University Press.

Barrett, W. (1958). *Irrational man: A study in existential philosophy*. New York: Anchor Books.

Bateman, A., & Fonagy, P. (2006). *Mentalization-based treatment for borderline personality disorder: A practical guide*. New York: Oxford University Press.

Beauchamp, T. I., & Childress, J. F. (2001). *Principles of medical ethics* (5th ed.). New York: Oxford University Press.

Beer, J. S. (2007). The importance of emotion–social cognition interactions for social functioning: Insights from the orbitofrontal cortex. In E. Harmon-Jones & P. Winkielman (Eds.), *Social neuroscience: Integrating biological and psychological explanations of social behavior* (pp. 15–30). New York: Guilford Press.

Benham, G., & Younger, J. (2008). Hypnosis and mind–body interactions. In M. R. Nash & A. J. Barnier (Eds.), *The Oxford handbook of hypnosis* (pp. 393–438). New York: Oxford University Press.

Berkman, L. F., Leo-Summers, L., & Horwitz, R. I. (1992). Emotional support and survival after myocardial infarction: A prospective population-based study of the elderly. *Annals of Internal Medicine, 117*, 1003–1009.

Blackham, H. J. (1952). *Six existentialist thinkers*. New York: Harper Torchbooks.

Blackner, K., & Wong, N. (1963). Four cases of autocastration. *Archives of General Psychiatry, 8*, 169–176.

Blass, D. M. (2007). A pragmatic approach to teaching psychiatry residents the assessment and treatment of religious patients. *Academic Psychiatry, 31*, 25–31.

Blazer, D. (2005). *The age of melancholy: Major depression and its social origins*. New York: Routledge.

Boehm, C. (1999). *Hierarchy in the forest*. Cambridge, MA: Harvard University Press.

Boisen, A. T. (1936/1962). *The exploration of the inner world: A study of mental disorder and religious experience*. New York: Harper & Brothers.

Boorstein, M. (2008, November 16). In Virginia, a powerful and polarizing pastor. *The Washington Post*, pp. A1, A10.

Bowlby, J. (1973). *Attachment and loss: Vol. 2. Separation: Anxiety and anger*. New York: Basic Books.

Brewer, M. B. (1991). The social self: On being the same and different at the same time. *Personality and Social Psychology Bulletin, 17*, 475–482.

Brewer, M. B. (1993). Social identity, distinctiveness, and in-group homogeneity. *Social Cognition, 11*, 150–164.

Brewer, M. B., & Miller, N. (1984). Beyond the contact hypothesis: Theoretical perspectives on desegregation. In N. Miller & M. B. Brewer (Eds.), *Groups in contact: The psychology of desegregation* (pp. 281–302). Orlando, FL: Academic Press.

Brewer, M. B., & Miller, N. (1988). Contact and cooperation: When do they work? In P. Katz & D. Taylor (Eds.), *Eliminating racism: Profiles in controversy* (pp. 315–326). New York: Plenum Press.

Brown, G. W., & Harris, T. (1978). *Social origins of depression*. London: Tavistock.

Buber, M. (1958). *I and thou* (2nd ed.). New York: Macmillan.

Bunyan, J. (1666/1987). *Grace abounding to the chief of sinners.* New York: Penguin. books.google.com

Busch, K. A., Fawcett, J., & Jacobs, D. G. (2003). Clinical correlates of inpatient suicide. *Journal of Clinical Psychiatry, 64,* 14–19.

Buss, D. M. (Ed.). (2005). *Handbook of evolutionary psychology.* New York: Wiley.

Cassell, E. J. (1991). *The nature of suffering and the goals of medicine.* New York: Oxford University Press.

Cattell, J. P., & Cattell, J. S. (1974). Depersonalization: Psychological and social perspectives. In S. Arieti (Ed.), *American handbook of psychiatry* (2nd ed., pp. 766–799). New York: Basic Books.

Central Intelligence Agency. (2008). *The world factbook.* Retrieved July 20, 2008, from *www.cia.gov/library/;publication/the-world-factbook.*

Chadwick, P. K. (2001). Sanity to supersanity to unsanity: A personal journey. In I. Clark (Ed.), *Psychosis and spirituality: Exploring the new frontier* (pp. 75–89). London: Whurr.

Chadwick, P. K. (2009). *Schizophrenia: The positive perspective.* New York: Routledge.

Chasin, R., Herzig, M., Roth, S., Chasin, L., Becker, C., & Stains, R. R., Jr. (1996). From diatribe to dialogue on divisive public issues: Approaches drawn from family therapy. *Mediation Quarterly, 13,* 1–19.

Ciechanowski, P. S., Katon, W. J., Russo, J. E., & Walker, E. A. (2001). The patient–provider relationship: Attachment theory and adherence to treatment in diabetes. *American Journal of Psychiatry, 158,* 29–35.

Claridge, G. (2001). Spiritual experience: Healthy psychoticism? In I. Clark (Ed.), *Psychosis and spirituality: Exploring the new frontier* (pp. 90–106). London: Whurr.

Clarke, I. (2001). Psychosis and spirituality: The discontinuity model. In I. Clark (Ed.), *Psychosis and spirituality: Exploring the new frontier* (pp. 129–142). London: Whurr.

Cobb, S. (2003). Fostering coexistence in identity-based conflicts: Toward a narrative approach. In A. Chayes & M. Minow *(Eds.), Imagine coexistence: Restoring humanity after violent ethnic conflict* (pp. 294–310). San Francisco: Jossey-Bass.

Crandall, C. S. (2000). Ideology and lay theories of stigma: The justification of stigmatization. In T. F. Heatherton, R. E. Kleck, M. R. Hebl, & J. G. Hull (Eds.), *The social psychology of stigma* (pp. 126–150). New York: Guilford Press.

Crippen, T., & Machalek, R. (1989). The evolutionary foundations of the religious life. *International Review of Sociology, 3,* 61–84.

Daly, M., & Wilson, M. (2005). Parenting and kinship. In D.M. Buss (Ed.), *The handbook of evolutionary psychology* (pp. 443–446). New York: Wiley.

Dapretto, M., Davies, M. S., Pfeifer, J. H., Scott, A. A., Sigman, M., Bookheimer, S. Y., et al. (2006). Understanding emotions in others: Mirror neuron dysfunction in children with autism spectrum disorders. *Nature Neuroscience, 9,* 28–30.

Davidson, J. R. T., & Connor, K. M. (2004). Treatment of anxiety disorders. In A. F. Schatzberg & C. B. Nemeroff (Eds.), *The American Psychiatric Publishing textbook of psychopharmacology* (3rd ed., pp. 913–934). Washington, DC: American Psychiatric Publishing.

Dawkins, R. (1989). *The selfish gene.* Oxford, UK: Oxford University Press.

de Figueiredo, J. M. (1993). Depression and demoralization: Phenomenological differences and research perspectives. *Comprehensive Psychiatry, 34,* 308–311.

de Quervain, D. J., Fischbacker, U., Treyer, V., Schellhammer, M., Schnyder, U., Buck, A., et al. (2004). The neural basis of altruistic punishment. *Science, 305,* 1254–1258.

Decety, J., & Grezes, J. (2006). The power of simulation: Imagining one's own and other's behavior. *Brain Research, 1079,* 4–14.

Decety, J., Jackson, P. L., Sommerville, J. A., Chaminade, T., & Meltzoff, A. N. (2004). The neural bases of cooperation and competition: An fMRI study. *NeuroImage, 23,* 744–751.

Devinsky, O., Feldmann, E., Burrowes, K., & Bromfield, E. (1989). Autoscopic phenomena with seizures. *Archives of Neurology, 46,* 1080–1088.

Dolan, M. (2008). Neurobiological disturbances in callous-unemotional youths. *American Journal of Psychiatry, 165,* 668–670.

Dostoevsky, F. (2004). *The idiot.* New York: Barnes & Nobles Classics. (Original work published 1869).

Dovidio, J. F., Major, B., & Crocker, J. (2000). Stigma: Introduction and overview. In T. F. Heatherton, R. E. Kleck, M. R. Hebl, & J. G. Hull (Eds.), *The social psychology of stigma* (pp. 1–3). New York: Guilford Press.

Eisen, J. L., & Rasmussen, S. A. (2002). Phenomenology of obsessive-compulsive disorder. In D. J. Stein & E. Hollander (Eds.), *The American Psychiatric Publishing textbook of anxiety disorders* (pp. 173–190). Washington, DC: American Psychiatric Publishing.

Eisenberger, N. I., Lieberman, M. D., & Williams, K. D. (2003). Does rejection hurt? An fMRI study of social exclusion. *Science, 302,* 290–292.

Ekman, P. (2003). *Emotions revealed* (2nd ed.). New York: Henry Holt.

Ell, K., Nishimoto, R., Mediansky, L., Mantell, J., & Hamovitch, M. (1992). Social relations, social support and survival among patients with cancer. *Journal of Psychosomatic Research, 36,* 531–541.

Erickson, M. H. (1980). On the nature of hypnosis. In E. Rossi (Ed.), *The collected works of Milton H. Erickson on hypnosis: Vol. I: The nature of hypnosis and suggestion* (pp. 1–132). New York: Irvington.

Erickson, M. H., & Erickson, E. M. (1980). The hypnotic induction of hallucinatory color vision followed by pseudonegative afterimages. In E. Rossi (Ed.), *The collected works of Milton H. Erickson on hypnosis: Vol. II: Hypnotic alteration of sensory, perceptual and psychophysiological processes* (pp. 5–10). New York: Irvington.

Fan, J., McCandliss, B. D., Sommer, T., Raz, A., & Posner, M. I. (2002). Testing the efficiency and independence of attentional networks. *Journal of Cognitive Neuroscience, 14,* 340–347.

Farrow, T. F. D., Zheng, Y., Wilkinson, I. D., Spence, S. A., Deakin, J. F., Tarrier, N., et al. (2001). Investigating the functional anatomy of empathy and forgiveness. *NeuroReport, 12,* 2433–2438.

Field, H. L., & Waldfogel, S. (1995). Severe ocular self-injury. *General Hospital Psychiatry, 17,* 224–227.

Fliessbach, K., Weber, B., Trautner, P., Dohmen, T., Sunde, U., Elger, C. E., et al. (2007). Social comparison affects reward-related brain activity in the human ventral striatum. *Science, 318,* 1305–1308.

Foucault, M. (1973). *The birth of the clinic: An archaeology of medical perception.* London: Tavistock.

Foucault, M. (1980). *Power/knowledge: Selected interviews and other writings.* New York: Pantheon.

Frank, J. D. (1961). *Persuasion and healing: A comparative study of psychotherapy* (1st ed.). Baltimore: Johns Hopkins University Press.

Frank, J. D., & Frank, J. B. (1991). *Persuasion and healing: A comparative study of psychotherapy* (3rd ed.). Baltimore: Johns Hopkins University Press.

Frost, R. (1915). *North of Boston.* New York: Henry Holt.

Gabbard, G. O. (2000). *Psychodynamic psychotherapy in clinical practice* (3rd ed.). Washington, DC: American Psychiatric Press.

Galanter, M. (1978). The "relief effect": A sociobiological model for neurotic distress and large-group therapy. *American Journal of Psychiatry, 135,* 588–591.

Galanter, M. (1999). *Cults: Faith, healing, and coercion* (2nd ed.). New York: Oxford University Press.

Galanter, M. (2005). *Spirituality and the healthy mind: Science, therapy, and the need for personal meaning.* New York: Oxford University Press.

Gennep, A. N. van (1909). *The rites of passage* (M. B. Vizedom & G. L. Caffee (Trans.). London: Routledge & Kegan Paul.

Giles, H., & Johnson, P. (1987). Ethnolinguistic identity theory: A social, psychological approach to language maintenance. *International Journal of the Sociology of Language, 68,* 69–99.

Gilman, T. T., & Marcuse, F. L. (1949). Animal hypnosis. *Psychological Bulletin, 46,* 151–165.

Gintis, H., Bowles, S., Boyd, R., & Fehr, E. (2003). Explaining altruistic behavior in humans. *Evolution and Human Behavior, 24,* 153–172.

Goffman, E. (1963). *Stigma: Notes on the management of spoiled identity.* New York: Simon & Schuster.

→ Goffman, E. (1967). *Interaction ritual: Essays on face-to-face behavior.* New York: Pantheon Books.

Griffith, J. L. (2006). Managing religious countertransference in clinical settings. *Psychiatric Annals, 36,* 196–204.

Griffith, J. L. (2010, May). Interviewing patients who hate or fear psychiatrists. Workshop presented at the 163rd Annual Meeting of the American Psychiatric Association, New Orleans, LA.

Griffith, J.L., & Dsouza, A. (in press). Demoralization and hope: Their role in clinical psychiatry and psychotherapy. In R. D. Alarcón, & J. B. Frank (Eds.), *The psychotherapy of hope: The legacy of Persuasion and Healing.* Baltimore: Johns Hopkins University Press.

Griffith, J. L., & Gaby, L. (2005). Brief psychotherapy at the bedside: Countering demoralization from medical illness. *Psychosomatics, 46,* 109–116.

References

Griffith, J. L., & Griffith, M. E. (1994). *The body speaks: Therapeutic dialogue* , *mind-body problems.* New York: Basic Books.

Griffith, J. L., & Griffith, M. E. (2002). *Encountering the sacred in psychotherapy: How* to talk with people about their spiritual lives. New York: Guilford Press.

Griffith, J. L., Griffith, M. E., Rains, J., Polles, A., Tingle, C., Krejmas, N., et al. (1995, October). *Analysis of intrapersonal self–God communications utilizing Structural Analysis of Social Behavior (SASB).* Paper presented at the annual meeting of the Society for the Scientific Study of Religion, St. Louis, MO.

Griffith, J. L., Polles, A., & Griffith, M. E. (1998). Pseudoseizures, families, & unspeakable dilemmas. *Psychosomatics, 39,* 144–153.

Griffiths, D. J. (1987). *Introduction to elementary particles.* New York: Wiley.

Grof, S., & Grof, C. (Eds.). (1989). *Spiritual emergency: When personal transformation becomes a crisis.* Los Angeles: Tarcher.

Groopman, J. (2004). *The anatomy of hope: How people prevail in the face of illness.* New York: Random House.

Gross, J. J. (2002). Emotional regulation: Affective, cognitive, and social consequences. *Psychophysiology, 39,* 281–291.

George Washington Institute for Spirituality and Health. (2008). *FICA spiritual history tool.* Retrieved June 5, 2008, from *www.gwish.org.*

Hamilton, A. (1967). Development of a rating scale for primary depressive illness. *British Journal of Social and Clinical Psychology, 6,* 278–296.

Hammarskjold, D. (1964). *Markings* (L. Sjoberg & W. H. Auden, Trans.). London: Faber and Faber.

Hardy, A. (1966). *The divine flame.* London: Collins.

Harris, J. C., & DeAngelis, C. D. (2008). The power of hope. *Journal of the American Medical Association, 300,* 2919–2920.

Heidegger, M. (1962). *Being and time.* New York: Harper & Row.

Heidegger, M. (1971). *On the way to language.* New York: Harper & Row.

Herzig, M., & Chasin, L. (2006). *Fostering dialogue across divides: A nuts and bolts guide from the Public Conversations Project.* Watertown, MA: Public Conversations Project.

Hibbard, J. H., & Pope, C. R. (1993). The quality of social roles as predictors of morbidity and mortality. *Social Science and Medicine, 36,* 217–225.

Hilgard, E. R., & Hilgard, J. R. (1983). *Hypnosis in the relief of pain* (rev. ed.). Los Altos, CA: William Kaufmann.

Hochschild, A. R. (1983). *The managed heart: Commercialization of human feeling.* Berkeley: University of California Press.

Hofbauer, R. K., Rainville, P., Duncan, G. H., & Bushnell, M. C. (2001). Cortical representation of the sensory dimension of pain. *Journal of Neurophysiology, 86,* 402–411.

Holmes, E. A., Brown, R. J., Mansell, W., Fearon, R. P., Hunter, E. C., Frasquilho, F., et al. (2005). Are there two qualitatively distinct forms of dissociation? A review and some clinical implications. *Clinical Psychology Review, 25,* 1–23.

Holy bible, revised standard version (1952). New York: Thomas Nelson.

Hood, R. W., Jr., Hill, P. C., & Spilka, B. (2009). *The psychology of religion: An empirical approach* (4th ed.). New York: Guilford Press.

Hood, R. W., Jr., Spilka, B., Hunsberger, B., & Gorsuch, R. (1996). *The psychology of religion: An empirical approach* (2nd ed.). New York: Guilford Press.

Horwitz, A. V., & Wakefield, J. C. (2007). *Loss of sadness: How psychiatry transformed normal sorrow into depressive disorder*. New York: Oxford University Press.

House, R. (2001). Psychopathology, psychosis and the kundalini: Postmodern perspectives on unusual subjective experience. In I. Clark (Ed.), *Psychosis and spirituality: Exploring the new frontier* (pp. 107–126). London: Whurr.

Hsu, M., Anen, C., & Quartz, S. R. (2008). The right and the good: Distributive justice and neural encoding of equity and efficiency. *Science, 320,* 1092–1995.

Hynes, C. A., Baird, A. A., & Grafton, S. T. (2006). Differential role of the orbital frontal lobe in emotional versus cognitive perspective-taking. *Neuropsychologia, 44,* 374–383.

Ilibagiza, I. (2006). *Left to tell: Discovering God amidst the Rwandan holocaust.* Carlsbad, CA: Hay House.

Jackson, J. W., & Smith, E. R. (1999). Conceptualizing social identity: A new framework and evidence for the impact of different dimensions. *Personality and Social Psychology Bulletin, 25,* 120–135.

Jackson, P. L., Rainville, P., & Decety, J. (2006). To what extent do we share the pain of others? Insight from the neural bases of pain empathy. *Pain, 125,* 5–9.

Jacobs, J., Kenis, G., Peeters, F., Derom, C., Vlietinck, R., & Os, J. V. (2006). Stress-related negative affectivity and genetically altered serotonin transporter function. *Archives of General Psychiatry, 63,* 989–996.

Jaspers, K. (1953). *The origin and goal of history.* New Haven, CT: Yale University Press.

Jewish Virtual Library. (n.d.). *Remarks by Heinrich Himmler: Speech of Reichsführer-SS Himmler, speaking to SS major-generals at Poznan, Poland, October 4, 1943.* Retrieved September 12, 2009, from *www. jewishvirtuallibrary.org/;source/Holocaust/himmler.html.*

Johnson, S., & Woolley, S. R. (2008). Emotionally focused couple therapy: An attachment based treatment. In G. Gabbard (Ed.), *The American Psychiatric Press textbook of psychotherapeutic treatments in psychiatry* (pp. 553–580). Washington, DC: American Psychiatric Press.

Josephson, A. M., & Peteet, J. R. (Eds.). (2004). *Handbook of spirituality and worldview in clinical practice.* Arlington, VA: American Psychiatric Publishing.

Jung, C. G. (1963). *Memories, dreams, reflections.* Recorded and edited by A. Jaffé. New York: Random House.

Kapuscinski, R. (2008). *The other.* New York: Verso.

Kearney, R. (1984). *Dialogues with five contemporary thinkers: Paul Ricoeur, Emmanuel Levinas, Herbert Marcuse, Stanislas Breton, Jacques Derrida.* New York: Manchester University Press.

Keysers, C. (2009, February). *From mirror neurons to empathy.* The 2009 Harvey Schein Lecture presented at the 38th Annual Meeting of the American Association of Directors of Psychiatry Residency Training, Tucson, AZ.

Kiehl, K. A. (2006). A cognitive neuroscience perspective on psychopathy: Evidence for paralimbic system dysfunction. *Psychiatry Research, 142,* 107–128.

Kierkegaard, S. (1968). *Fear and trembling and sickness unto death.* (W. Lowrie, Trans.). Princeton, NJ: Princeton University Press.

Kihlstrom, J. F. (2008). The domain of hypnosis, revisited. In M. R. Nash & A. J. Barnier (Eds.), *The Oxford handbook of hypnosis* (pp. 21–52). New York: Oxford University Press.

Kildahl, J. P. (1972). *The psychology of speaking in tongues.* New York: Harper & Row.

King-Casas, B., Tomlin, D., Anen, C., Camerer, C. F., Quartz, S. R., & Montague, P. R. (2005). Getting to know you: Reputation and trust in a two-person economic exchange. *Science, 308,* 78–83.

Kingdon, D., Siddle, R., & Rathod, S. (2001). Spirituality, psychosis and the development of 'normalising rationales.' In I. Clark (Ed.), *Psychosis and spirituality: Exploring the new frontier* (pp. 222–235). London: Whurr.

Kingdon, D. G., & Turkington, D. (1991). Preliminary report: The use of cognitive behaviour therapy with a normalizing rationale in schizophrenia. *Journal of Nervous and Mental Disease, 179,* 207–211.

Kingdon, D. G., & Turkington, D. (1994). *Cognitive-behavioral therapy of schizophrenia.* New York: Guilford Press.

Kirkpatrick, L. A. (2005). *Attachment, evolution, and the psychology of religion.* New York: Guilford Press.

Kleinman, A. (1988). *Rethinking psychiatry: From cultural category to personal experience.* New York: Free Press.

Kleinman, A. (2006). *What really matters: Living a moral life amidst uncertainty and danger.* New York: Oxford University Press.

Kleinman, A., Eisenberg, L., & Good, B. (1978). Culture, illness, and care: Clinical lessons from anthropologic and cross-cultural research. *Annals of Internal Medicine, 88,* 251–258.

Klemm, W. R. (2001). Behavioral arrest: In search of the neural control system. *Progress in Neurobiology, 65,* 453–471.

Klempner, M. (2006). *The heart has reasons: Holocaust rescuers and their stories of courage.* Cleveland, OH: Pilgrim Press.

Koenig, H. G. (Ed.). (1998). *Handbook of religion and mental health.* Boston: Academic Press.

Koenig, H. G., Cohen, H. J., George, L. K., Hays, J. C., Larson, D. B., & Blazer, D. G. (1997). Attendance at religious services, interleukin-6, and other biological parameters of immune function in older adults. *International Journal of Psychiatry in Medicine, 27,* 233–250.

Krebs, D. (2005). The evolution of morality. In D. M. Buss (Ed.), *The handbook of evolutionary psychology* (pp. 747–771). Hoboken, NJ: Wiley.

Krishna, G. (1971). *Kundalini: The evolutionary energy in man.* Berkeley, CA: Shambhala.

Kroger, W. S. (1977). *Clinical and experimental hypnosis* (2nd ed.). Philadelphia: Lippincott.

Kurland, J. A., & Gaulin, S. J. C. (2005). Cooperation and conflict among kin. In

D. M. Buss, (Ed.), *The handbook of evolutionary psychology* (pp. 447–482). New York: Wiley.

Kurzban, R., & Leary, M. R. (2001). Evolutionary origins of stigmatization: The functions of social exclusion. *Psychological Bulletin, 127,* 187–208.

Kushner, A.W. (1967). Two cases of autocastration due to religious delusions. *British Journal of Medical Psychology, 40,* 293–298.

Lamm C., Batson, D., & Decety J. (2007). The neural substrate of human empathy: Effects of perspective taking and cognitive appraisal. *Journal of Cognitive Neuroscience, 19,* 42–58.

Lazare, A. (1999, March 13). *Shame and humiliation in training and life.* Keynote address presented at the 28th Annual Meeting of the American Association of Directors of Psychiatric Residency Training, Santa Monica, CA.

Lazare, A. (2004). *On apology.* New York: Oxford University Press.

Lerner, M.J. (1980). *Belief in a just world.* New York: Plenum Press.

Levi, P. (1988). *The drowned and the saved.* New York: Vintage Books.

Levi, P. (1996). *Survival in Auschwitz.* New York: Simon & Schuster. (Original work published 1958)

Levinas, E. (1961). *Totality and infinity* (A. Lingis, trans.). Pittsburgh: Duquesne University Press.

Levinas, E. (1997). *Otherwise than being* (or *beyond essence*) (A. Lingis, Trans.). Pittsburgh: Duquesne University Press. (Original work published 1981)

Lieberman, M. D. (2007). The X- and C-systems: The neural basis of automatic and controlled social cognition. In E. Harmon-Jones & P. Winkielman (Eds.), *Social neuroscience: Integrating biological and psychological explanations of social behavior* (pp. 290–315). New York: Guilford Press.

Lifton, R. J. (1986). *The Nazi doctors.* New York: Basic Books.

Lukoff, D. (2007). Visionary spiritual experiences. *Southern Medical Journal, 100,* 635–641.

Malcolm, N. (1998). *Kosovo: A short history.* New York: New York University Press.

Maldonado, J. R., & Spiegel, D. (2008a). Dissociative disorders. In A. Tasman, J. Kay, A. Lieberman, M. B. First, & M. Maj (Eds.), *Psychiatry* (3rd ed., pp. 1558–1577). West Sussex, UK: Wiley-Blackwell.

Maldonado, J. R., & Spiegel, D. (2008b). Hypnosis. In A. Tasman, J. Kay, J. A. Lieberman, M. B. First, & M. Maj (Eds.), *Psychiatry* (3rd ed., pp. 1982–2026). West Sussex, UK: Wiley-Blackwell.

Marek, G., & Duman, R. S. (2002). Neural circuitry and signaling in depression. In B. B. Kaplan & R. P. Hammer (Eds.), *Brain circuitry and signaling in psychiatry: Basic science and clinical implications (pp. 153–178). Washington: American Psychiatric Pub.*

Maturana, H., & Varela, F. J. (1992). *The tree of knowledge: The biological roots of human understanding.* Boston: Shambhala.

McClenon, J. (1997). Shamanic healing, human evolution, and the origin of religion. *Journal for the Scientific Study of Religion, 36,* 345–354.

McDargh, J. (1983). *Psychoanalytic object relations theory and the study of religion.* New York: University Press of America.

McFarlane, A. C. (2002). Phenomenology of posttraumatic stress disorder. In D. J. Stein & E. Hollander (Eds.), *The American Psychiatric Publishing textbook of anxiety disorders* (pp. 359–373). Washington, DC: American Psychiatric Publishing.

Mechanic, D. (1986). Role of social factors in health and well being: Biopsychosocial model from a social perspective. *Integrative Psychiatry, 4,* 2–11.

Meissner, W. W. (1984). *Psychoanalysis and religious experience.* New Haven, CT: Yale University Press.

Meissner, W. W. (1987). Projection and projective identification. In J. Sandler (Ed.), *Projection, identification and projective identification* (pp. 27–49). Madison, CT: International Universities Press.

Merton, T. (1969). *Comtemplative prayer.* New York: Herder and Herder.

Mesulam, M.-M. (2000). *Principles of behavioral and cognitive neurology* (2nd ed.). New York: Oxford University Press.

Miernat, M., & Dovidio, J. F. (2000). Stigma and stereotypes. In T. F. Heatherton, R. E. Kleck, M. R. Hebl, & J. G. Hull (Eds.), *The social psychology of stigma.* New York: Guilford Press.

Milamaaria, V., Saarela, M. V., Hlushchuk, Y., Williams, A. C. d. C., Shurmann, M., Kalso, E., & Hari, R. (2007). The compassionate brain: Humans detect intensity of pain from another's face. *Cerebral Cortex, 17,* 230–237.

Miller, W. R. (Ed.). (1999). *Integrating spirituality into treatment: Resources for practitioners.* Washington, DC: American Psychological Association.

Mills, N. (2001). The experience of fragmentation in psychosis: Can mindfulness help? In I. Clark (Ed.), *Psychosis and spirituality: Exploring the new frontier* (pp. 211–221). London: Whurr.

Mithen, S. (1996). *The prehistory of the mind: A search for the origins of art, religion and science.* London: Thames & Hudson.

Monk, R. (1991). *Ludwig Wittgenstein: The duty of genius.* New York: Penguin Books.

Mookadam, F., & Arthur, H. M. (2004). Social support and its relationship to morbidity and mortality after acute myocardial infarction: Systematic review. *Archives of Internal Medicine, 164,* 1514–1518.

Morse, D. (2009, March 29). Death opens doors on group: Ministry members charged in Baltimore after baby's body is found. *Washington Post,* pp. C1, C4.

Neuberg, S. L., Smith, D. M., & Asher, T. (2000). Why people stigmatize: Toward a biocultural framework. In T. F. Heatherton, R. E. Kleck, M. R. Hebl, & J. G. Hull (Eds.), *The social psychology of stigma.* New York: Guilford Press.

Norris, C. J., & Cacioppo, J. T. (2007). I know how you feel: Social and emotional information processing in the brain. In E. Harmon-Jones & P.A. Winkielman (Eds.), *Social neuroscience: Integrating biological and psychological explanations of social behavior* (pp. 84–105). New York: Guilford Press.

Noss, J.B. (1963). *Man's religions* (3rd ed.). New York: Macmillan.

Oberman, L. M., & Ramachandran, V. S. (2007). The simulating mind: The role of the mirror neuron system and simulation in the social and communicative deficits of autism spectrum disorders. *Psychological Bulletin, 133,* 310–327.

Ochsner, K. N. (2007). How thinking controls feeling: A social cognitive neuroscience approach. In E. Harmon-Jones & P.A. Winkielman (Eds.), *Social neuro-*

science: Integrating biological and psychological explanations of social behavior (pp. 106–136). New York: Guilford Press.

Ochsner, K. N., Bunge, S. A., Gross, J. J., & Gabrieli, J. D. E. (2002). Rethinking feelings: An fMRI study of the cognitive regulation of emotion. *Journal of Cognitive Neuroscience, 14*, 1215–1229.

Orwell, G. (1949). *Nineteen eighty-four. A novel.* New York: Harcourt, Brace.

Papp, L. A., & Kleber, M. S. (2002). Phenomenology of generalized anxiety disorder. In D. J. Stein & E. Hollander (Eds.), *The American Psychiatric Publishing textbook of anxiety disorders* (pp. 109–118). Washington, DC: American Psychiatric Publishing.

Pargament, K. I. (1997). *The psychology of religion and coping: Theory, research, practice.* New York: Guilford Press.

Pargament, K. I. (2007). *Spiritually integrated psychotherapy.* New York: Guilford Press.

Pargament, K. I., Koenig, H. G., Tarakeshwar, N. (2001). Religious struggle as a predictor of mortality among medically ill elderly patients. *Archives of Internal Medicine, 161*, 1881–1885.

Pargament, K. I., Koenig, H. G., Tarakeshwar, N., & Hahn, J. (2004). Religious coping methods as predictors of psychological, physical and spiritual outcomes among medically-ill elderly patients: A longitudinal study. *Journal of Health Psychology, 9*, 1713–1730.

Parker, L. (1980). *We let our son die: A parent's search for truth.* Irvine, CA: Harvest House.

Perdue, C. W., Dovidio, J. F., Gurtman, M. B., & Tyler, R. B. (1990). Us and them: Social categorization and the process of intergroup bias. *Journal of Personality and Social Psychology, 59*, 475–486.

Peterson, R. (1986). *Everyone is right: A new look at comparative religion and its relation to science.* Marina del Ray, CA: DeVorss.

Polkinghorne, D. E. (1988). *Narrative knowing and the human sciences.* Albany: State University of New York Press.

Pollack, M. H., Smoller, J. W., Otto, M. W., Scott, E. L., & Rosenbaum, J. F. (2002). Phenomenology of panic disorder. In D. J. Stein & E. Hollander (Eds.), *The American Psychiatric Publishing textbook of anxiety disorders* (pp. 237–246). Washington: American Psychiatric Publishing.

Polles, A., Rains, J., Tingle, C., Krejmas, N., Griffith, J., Griffith, M. E., et al. (1993, October). *Characterizing God-self relationships.* Paper presented at the annual meeting of the Society for the Scientific Study of Religion, Raleigh, NC.

Posner, M. I., & Peterson, S. E. (1990). The attention system of the human brain. *Annual Review of Neuroscience, 13*, 25–42.

Post, J. M. (2007). *The mind of the terrorist.* New York: Palgrave Macmillan.

Pratto, F. (1999). The puzzle of continuing group inequality: Piecing together psychological, social, and cultural forces in social dominance theory. In M. P. Zanna (Ed.), *Advances in experimental social psychology* (Vol. 312, pp. 191–263). San Diego: Academic Press.

Pratto, F., Sidanius, J., Stallworth, L. M., & Malle, B. F. (1994). Social dominance orientation: A personality variable predicting social and political attitudes. *Journal of Personality and Social Psychology, 67,* 741–763.

Price, D. D., Barrell, J. J., & Rainville, P. (2002). Integrating experiential-phenomenonological methods and neuroscience to study neural mechanisms of pain and consciousness. *Consciousness and Cognition, 11,* 593–608.

Puchalski, C. M., Larson, D., & Lu, D. (2001). Spirituality in psychiatry residency training programs. *International Review of Psychiatry, 13,* 131–138.

Pulleyblank Coffey, E. (2007). *Blowing on embers.* Tamarac, FL: Llumina Press.

Rainville, P., Duncan, G. H., Price, D. D., Carrier, B., & Bushnell, M. C. (1997). Pain affect encoded in human anterior cingulate but not somatosensory cortex. *Science, 277,* 968–971.

Rainville, P., Hofbauer, R. K., Bushnell, M. C., Duncan, G. H., & Price, D. D. (1999). Dissociation of sensory and affective dimensions of pain using hypnotic modulation. *Pain, 82,* 159–171.

Rainville, P., Hofbauer, R. K., Bushnell, M. C., Duncan, G. H., & Price, D. D. (2002). Hypnosis modulates the activity in cerebral structures involved in the regulation of consciousness. *Journal of Cognitive Neuroscience, 14*(Suppl.), 887–901.

Ramsland, K. (2005). *Andrea Yates: Ill or evil?* Retrieved September 28, 2009, from www.trutv.com/library/crime/notorious_murders/women/andrea_yates/.

Rauch, S. L., Shin, L. M., & Phelps, E. A. (2006). Neurocircuitry models of post-traumatic stress disorder and extinction: Human neuroimaging research—past, present, and future. *Biological Psychiatry, 60,* 376–382.

Ridley, M. (1996). *The origins of virtue: Human instincts and the evolution of cooperation.* New York: Viking.

Rizzolatti, G., & Craighero, L. (2004). The mirror-neuron system. *Annual Review of Neuroscience, 27,* 169–192.

Rizzuto, A.-M. (1979). *The birth of the living God: A psychoanalytic study.* Chicago: University of Chicago Press.

Robins, R. S., & Post, J. (1997). *Political paranoia: The psychopolitics of hatred.* New Haven, CT: Yale University Press.

Rothschild, B. (2000). *The body remembers: The psychophysiology of trauma and trauma treatment.* New York: Norton.

Rothschild, B. (2003). *The body remembers casebook: Unifying methods and models in the treatment of trauma and PTSD.* New York: Norton.

Ruby, P., & Decety, J. (2004). How would *you* feel versus how do you think *she* would feel? A neuroimaging study of perspective-taking with social emotions. *Journal of Cognitive Neuroscience, 16,* 988–999.

Sartre, J. P. (1962). *Nausea.* New York: New Directions. (Original work published 1938)

Scarnati, R., Madry, M., Wise, A., & Moore, H.D. (1991). Religious beliefs and practices among the most-dangerous psychiatric inmates. *Forensic Reports, 4,* 1–16.

Schneider, D. J. (2004). *The psychology of stereotyping.* New York: Guilford Press.

Seitz, R., Nickel, J., & Azari, N. P. (2006). Functional modularity of the medial prefrontal cortex: Involvement in human empathy. *Neuropsychology, 20,* 743–751.

Shamay-Tsoory, S. G., Tomer, R., Berger, B. D., Goldsher, D, & Aharon-Peretz, J.

(2005). Impaired "affective theory of mind" is associated with right ventrome-dial prefrontal damage. *Cognitive and Behavioral Neurology, 18,* 55–67.

Shea, S. (2002). *The practical art of suicide assessment.* Hoboken, NJ: Wiley.

Shepard, G. M. (1994). *Neurobiology* (3rd ed.). New York: Oxford University Press.

Shimamura, A. P. (2000). The role of the prefrontal cortex in dynamic filtering. *Psychobiology, 28,* 207–218.

Sidanius, J., & Pratto, F. (1999). *Social dominance: An intergroup theory of hierarchy and oppression.* New York: Cambridge University Press.

Siegel, D. J. (1999). *The developing mind: Toward a neurobiology of interpersonal experience.* New York: Guilford Press.

Siegel, D. J. (2007). *The mindful brain: Reflection and attunement in the cultivation of well-being.* New York: Norton.

Simeon, D., & Abugel, J. (2006). *Feeling unreal: Depersonalization disorder and the loss of the self.* New York: Oxford University Press.

Singer, T., Seymour, B., O'Doherty, J., Kaube, H., Dolan, R. J., & Frith, C. D. (2004). Empathy for pain involves the affective but not sensory components of pain. *Science, 303,* 1157–1162.

Singer, T., Seymour, B., O'Doherty, J. P., Stephan, K. E., Dolan, R. J., & Frith, C. D. (2006). Empathic neural responses are modulated by the perceived fairness of others. *Nature, 439,* 466–469.

Singer, T. S. (1995). *Cults in our midst: The hidden menace in our everyday lives.* San Francisco: Jossey-Bass.

Slakter, E. (Ed). (1987). *Countertransference.* Northvale, NJ: Jason Aronson.

Slavney, P. R. (1999). Diagnosing demoralization in consultation psychiatry. *Psychosomatics, 40,* 325–329.

Sloan, R. P. (2006). *Blind faith: The unholy alliance of religion and medicine.* New York: St. Martin's Press.

Sloan, R. P. (2007, August 9). *First, do no evangelizing.* Retrieved September 30, 2007, from www.newsweek.washingtonpost.com/unfaith/guestvoices/2007/08/should_the_medical_care_you.html.

Sloan, R. P., Bagiella, E., VandeCreek, L., & Poulos, P. (2000). Should physicians prescribe religious activities? *New England Journal of Medicine, 342,* 1913–1916.

Snyder, C. R. (2000a). Genesis: The birth and growth of hope. In C. R. Snyder (Ed.), *Handbook of hope: Theory, measures, and applications* (pp. 25–38). New York: Academic Press.

Snyder, C. R. (2000b). Hypothesis: There is hope. In C.R. Snyder (Ed.), *Handbook of hope: Theory, measures, and applications* (pp. 3–24). New York: Academic Press.

Snyder, C. R., & Taylor, J. D. (2000). Hope as a common factor across psychotherapy approaches: A lesson from dodo's verdict. In C. R. Snyder (Ed.), *Handbook of hope: Theory, measures, and applications* (pp. 89–108). New York: Academic Press.

Sperry, L., & Shafranske, E.P. (Eds.). (2005). *Spiritually oriented psychotherapy.* Washington, DC: American Psychological Association.

Spiegel, D. (2008). Intelligent design or designed intelligence? Hypnotizability as neurobiological adaptation. In M. R. Nash & A. J. Barnier (Eds.), *The Oxford hand-*

book of hypnosis: Theory, research and practice (pp. 179–200). New York: Oxford University Press.

Stein, D. J. (2000). The neurobiology of evil: Psychiatric perspectives on perpetrators. *Ethnicity and Health, 5,* 303–315.

Stuart, S., & Noyes, R. (1999). Attachment and interpersonal communication in somatization. *Psychosomatics, 40,* 34–43.

Sumner, W. G. (1907). *Folkways.* Boston: Ginn.

Sweetingham, L. (2006, December 31). *Andrea Yates case: Expert: Andrea Yates believed she was battling Satan when she drowned her children.* Retrieved September 28, 2009, from edition.cnn.com/2007/US/law/12/11/court.archive.yates7.

Tajfel, H. (Ed.). (1979). *Differentiation between social groups: Studies in the social psychology of intergroup relations.* New York: Academic Press.

Tajfel, H. (Ed.). (1981). *Human groups and social categories: Studies in social psychology.* New York: Cambridge University Press.

Tajfel, H. (Ed.). (1982). *Social identity in intergroup relations.* New York: Cambridge University Press.

Taylor, S. E., & Gonzaga, G. C. (2007). Affiliative responses to stress: A social neuroscience model. In E. Harmon-Jones & P. Winkielman (Eds.), *Social neuroscience: Integrating biological and psychological explanations of social behavior* (pp. 290–315). New York: Guilford Press.

Tobert, N. (2001). The polarities of consciousness. In I. Clark (Ed.), *Psychosis and spirituality: Exploring the new frontier* (pp. 29–52). London: Whurr.

Tucker, D. M., Luu, P., & Derryberry, D. (2005). Love hurts: The evolution of empathic concern through the encephalization of nociceptive capacity. *Development and Psychopathology, 17,* 699–713.

Turner, J. C. (1987). *Rediscoverying the social group: A self-categorization theory.* Oxford, UK: Blackwell.

Turner, J. C. (1991). *Social influence.* Pacific Grove, CA: Brooks/Cole.

Turner, J. C. (1999). Some current issues in research on social identity and self- categorization theories. In N. Ellemers, R. Spears, & B. Doosje (Eds.), *Social identity: Context, commitment, content* (pp. 6–34). Oxford, UK: Blackwell.

Turner, V. (1969). *The ritual process: Structure and anti-structure.* Ithaca, NY: Cornell University Press.

Turner, V. (1974). *Dramas, fields, and metaphors: Symbolic action in human society.* Ithaca, NY: Cornell University Press.

Turner, V. (1982). *From ritual to theatre: The human seriousness of play.* Baltimore, MD: PAJ Publications/Johns Hopkins University Press.

Uchino, B. N., Holt-Lunstad, J., Uno, D., Campo, R., & Reblin, M. (2007). The social neuroscience of relationships: An examination of health relevant pathways. In E. Harmon-Jones & P. Winkielman (Eds.), *Social neuroscience: Integrating biological and psychological explanations of social behavior* (pp. 474–492). New York: Guilford Press.

Volkan, V. (2006). *Killing in the name of identity: A study of bloody conflicts.* Charlottesville, VA: Pitchstone Publishing.

Vygotsky, L. (1986). *Thought and language.* Cambridge, MA: MIT Press.

Wade, A. (1997). Small acts of living: Everyday resistance to violence and other forms of oppression. *Contemporary Family Therapy, 19*, 23–39.

Watkins, M. (1986). *Invisible guests: The development of imaginal dialogues.* Hillsdale, NJ: Analytic Press.

Waxler-Morrison, N., Hislop, T. G., Mears, B., & Kan L. (1991). Effects of social relationships on survival for women with breast cancer: a prospective study. *Social Science and Medicine, 33*, 177–83.

Weihs, K. L., Enright, T. M., & Simmens, S. J. (2008). Close relationships and emotional processing predict decreased mortality in women with breast cancer: Preliminary evidence. *Psychosomatic Medicine, 70*, 117–124.

Weingarten K. (1995). Attending to absence. *Journal of Feminist Family Therapy, 7*, 1–5.

Weingarten, K. (2003). *Common shock: Witnessing violence every day—How we are harmed, how we can heal.* New York: Dutton Press.

Weingarten, K. (2007). Hope in a time of global despair. In C. Flaskas, I. McCarthy, & J. Sheehan (Eds.), *Hope and despair in narrative and family therapy: Adversity, forgiveness and reconciliation* (pp. 13–23). New York: Routledge.

Weingarten, K. (2010). Reasonable hope: Construct, clinical applications, and supports. *Family Process, 49*, 5–25.

Weisberg, R., & Clark, D. (Producers). (1988). *We let our son die* [Television program]. Los Angeles: Dick Clark Productions.

White, M. (1995). *Re-authoring lives: Interviews and essays.* Adelaide, South Australia: Dulwich Centre Publications.

White, M. (2007). *Maps of narrative practice.* New York: Norton.

Wikipedia. (2006). *Andrea Yates.* Retrieved June 24, 2009, from *en.wikipedia.org/wiki/Andrea_Yates.*

Wikipedia. (2009). *Heaven's gate (religious group).* Retrieved September 16, 2009, from *en.wikipedia.org/wiki/Heaven's_Gate_(religious_group).*

Wilson, E. O. (2004). *On human nature: Revised edition.* Cambridge, MA: Harvard University Press.

Wilson, W. P. (1998). Religion and psychoses. In H. G. Koenig (Ed.), *Handbook of religion and mental health* (pp. 161–174). San Diego: Academic Press.

Winnicott, D. W. (1949). Hate in the counter-transference. *International Journal of Psychoanalysis, 30*, 69–74.

Winnicott, D. W. (1965). *The maturational processes and the facilitating environment.* New York: International Universities Press.

Yalom, I. (1989). *Love's executioner and other tales of psychotherapy.* New York: Basic Books.

Zinnbauer, B. J., & Pargament, K. I. (2005). Religiousness and spirituality. In R. F. Paloutzian & C. L. Park (Eds.), *Handbook of the psychology of religion and spirituality* (pp. 21–42). New York: Guilford Press.

Zinner, J. (2008). Psychodynamic couples therapy: An object relations approach. In G. Gabbard (Ed.), *The American Psychiatric Publishing textbook of psychotherapeutic treatments in psychiatry* (pp. 581–602). Washington, DC: American Psychiatric Publishing.

Index